Feminine Wisdom: Rise of a New Creation

"helping women regain hope and health, when faced with Fertility Challenges."

Body, Mind & Soul Medicine to heal imbalances in Fertility & Reproductive System.

Dr. Leonor Murciano-Chen

The Real Medicine is the healing that comes by honoring our Truth of the Divine within. As women, that deep wisdom is weaved innately in the very soul of our being; in the soul of the Feminine.

.

True Healing occurs when we accept who we are and what we carry from the Divine.

We are the Love…. The treasure is Within…

Our Essence is through Feminine Principle…

Honor her and we honor our selves.

Do you think you are a small star,
while the whole universe
is contained within you?
Shaykh Muhammad Sa'id al-Jamal ar-Rifai as-Shadhuli

Written by
Dr. Leonor Murciano-Chen, OMD
Nourishing Women Corp.
NourishingWomenCenter.com

Published by Nura Light Publishing
October 2010

Patient Experiences

Patient 1:

I began acupuncture therapy as a complement to my fertility treatment as it was highly recommended to increase my fertility chance for success. At my first appointment with Dr. Murciano, I was impressed by the holistic way she viewed my symptoms and infertility issues and by how the therapy approached the body as a whole, unified system. Her positive outlook and her determination that my issues were treatable and could be resolved through acupuncture were very encouraging. I began acupuncture therapy twice a week throughout my fertility treatment and truly believe that it led to the success of the treatment and the healthy progression of my subsequent pregnancy. During the first trimester of my pregnancy, acupuncture helped relieve my nausea, increase my energy and calm my mind. Dr. Murciano always greeted me with a smile and seemed to truly care about how things were going in my life. Our sessions focused not only on treating my infertility and pregnancy but also balancing other aspects of my life, such as fatigue and stress. I have many thanks to give to Dr. Murciano for everything she has done for me and highly recommend acupuncture therapy to any couple experiencing infertility.

Patient: Claudia

Patient 2:

I came to Dr. Murciano for acupuncture sessions in an attempt to increase the success fullness of IVF. I was desperate to have a baby and had read research that showed that acupuncture greatly increased the likelihood of conceiving and having a child. At the time of our first session, I was struggling with overwhelming anxiety and fear. I was experiencing panic attacks on a daily basis, severe insomnia, and unbearable depression. Fear of the unknown was ruling my life. During our initial consult, Dr. Murciano recommended healing sessions and Chinese medicine in addition to the acupuncture. Thus began this chapter of healing in my life. My anxiety and depression symptoms have significantly decreased, I rarely experience panic attacks, I sleep much better, and overall have more faith in myself. I am learning to love myself and trust more deeply that I am exactly where I am supposed to be.
Patient: C.K. Florida

Patient 3:

A couple of years ago, at the age of 34, I was told that I have the FSH values of a woman in her 40's. This condition is called premature ovarian failure. In the past, I have had FSH values of 14.7, 7.8, and most recently a 9.1 in October of 2005. (A woman who is 35 is supposed to have an FSH of 7 or lower.) Last October, my reproductive endocrinologist wanted me to do an IVF cycle right away, warning me that if my FSH got too high, that he would not be able to help me. My husband and I preferred to do the cycle about five months later but were concerned that my FSH might get too high if we waited, and there is no solution in western medicine to treat high FSH. That is why I turned to eastern medicine and Dr. Murciano-Luna for help. After only six weeks of acupuncture and herbs, my reproductive endocrinologist was very surprised and happy for me when my latest FSH came back as a 5.2. To my knowledge, this is the best value in my recorded history and we have been approved to start the IVF cycle.

Patient: Stephanie

Patient 4:

Pure Love. The kind of love that fills up your body and heart, and brings tears of happiness to your eyes. This is what I experience every day I hold my daughter. I never knew how to allow this kind of love and happiness in my life, until I met Dr. Murciano.

My story is like many women, trouble conceiving and willing to try anything. After countless surgeries for endometriosis, and terrible monthly pain, acupuncture seemed like a logical more holistic approach. However, my experience was more than just needles. Dr. Murciano taught me how to care for my body, how foods affected my health, and made me look at my emotions, and where sadness and resentment stemmed from.

After more infertility treatments, and several sessions of acupuncture, it was time to turn to IVF. At this point, I was at my breaking point emotionally, and turned to healings to help me get through the cycle. This is where Dr. Murciano's work literally changed my life. I know that sounds like a cliché, but she helped me heal years of pain and resentment. She taught me how to let the light in, live my life guided by love, and to not make decisions out of fear. Basically just "be".

The Healing Meditations and Chinese Medicine started me on a lifelong journey, one that has resulted in the most important love….the love of myself and my child. After 5 years of trying, I became a mother. I had a 10% chance of In Vitro working. We made ONE embryo—a miracle!! I truly believe Lila wouldn't be in our lives if it wasn't for Dr. Murciano's compassion, love and understanding. Thank you for this amazing gift, I can't wait to continue to grow with your guidance.

Live Love!

Kristen Hewitt (Lila's mommy!)

Dedication

I dedicate this book to the Divine Presence of the Feminine that lies within our very essence, in the very soul of Women. I am grateful to be a part in the gradual integration of this essence in our World.

I dedicate this book to everyone that has touched my life and has been a mirror for me, sharing a glimpse of the beauty, depth, wisdom as well as many other divine qualities that we all carry.

For all my teachers, academically and spiritually, I thank you, for you have given me a great gift of the Truth, and led me to unspeakable territories. For all my patients, I thank all of you for allowing me to serve each and every one of you, as you provided me with an arena in which to explore the mysteries of our deeper selves and the beauty of the feminine soul.

I am also extremely grateful for all those Teachers and Healers infusing the soul back in to the heart of the world and guiding others into the healing of their being, one person at a time.

I most graciously thank my husband for his understanding, patience and willingness to meet me wherever I'm at. And I also thank my four girls; Kaelyn, Erin, Mia and Meilin, for their generosity of giving up a little of "mom" to share with the world, (whether they wanted to or not). For these little beings (or not so little anymore) are my true teachers in my walking.

And last but certainly not least, I want to thank my mother, for always being the one willing to step out into uncharted territory and inspire me to continue to search for Truth until I reached it.

Preface

What happens to us when the very thing that defines us as Women, our reproductive system seems to be malfunctioning and experiencing some level of disorder perhaps even disease? What happens when what we think others define us by, within our bodies, is somehow defective, and what does that say about us as women? Does that make us less of a woman, or defective in some way? Do we then, identify ourselves with being dysfunctional, maybe even unworthy or as a helpless victim?

The condition of our physical body is a reflection of deep unconscious feelings. How we feel about ourselves as women is generally reflected in our being, and the reproductive area is symbolic of these deeper feelings. If we are experiencing disorders buried in this part of our physical body, we can serve ourselves well by exploring our deep seated feelings and centuries old attitudes about the meaning of womanhood.

In order to heal our reproductive system from such diseases as endometriosis, infertility, and polycystic ovaries; to name a few, we must ask ourselves these questions and open ourselves to the full potential of the Feminine and discover for ourselves what that is.

Introduction

A desperate yearning, a quiet loneliness, hopelessness and a constant river of disappointment, coupled with the shadow land of shame and confusion depicts our issues with Fertility. Women suffer in silence, as they watch their bodies, month after month, year after year; betray their greatest gift given to them at birth. As they are denied this innate ability of fertility, that has defined their very essence since the beginning of time; they unavoidably deal with the exasperating feelings of anger, rage, sadness, and defeat. Not understanding why they have been chosen by life, to receive such a cruel punishment, they seek and search far and wide in order to break free from the dark cloud that seems to lurk over them.

Deep in their hearts their longing to experience reproductive health, becomes bigger than life itself. But explanations seem scarce and victories are few. Adding to this colossal of turbulence is the underlying shame of having been branded with a reproductive disorder. Thus, the disorder involving the reproductive system is not something that can be discussed openly among friends and society, without a subtle judgment of disgrace. This underlining shadow of shame creeps in to every thought and becomes infused in the very definition of their being. They start to feel less than their average female counterpart, tainted somehow, as if there was an unspoken curse and they were reluctantly living in it.

Our society, steeped in old beliefs, serves to lock this foundation in place by supporting women's feelings of failure rather than their true image of beauty and holiness. Seemingly innocent, a woman's own consciousness continues to contribute to the undulating shame that seems to be part of this fall from grace.

Awareness, however, is the foundation on the yellow brick road of hope that can carry us out of this darkness and into the light. Once we understand, we do not need to look back and stay stuck in our old ways. In the search for health options, as with any disorder in our bodies, we run in to ourselves. We run into the very essential questions that trigger our quest of who we are and what our body is experiencing. Once the conventional medical treatments have all been utilized without delivering the desired results, we are forced to ask these questions about ourselves as women, and as human beings.

Our continued sanity requires that we search within for answers and face some of the deeper questions of existence that most of us usually avoid. These questions undoubtedly define ourselves outside of our limiting beliefs and redefine ourselves as Women, perhaps with a view that includes all of our existing challenges by definition. Perhaps the new view will incorporate all of our experiences and also bring us closer to our wholeness, leaving us feeling more of ourselves, rather than less. Perhaps what we may uncover is that we have more happiness, more joy, more life than we have been believing that we can have and perhaps our new awareness of who and what we are, will free us to be all that we really are; a Divine Jewel.

Crossing the Bridge to Discovery

A new discovery can be found through this pinhole of darkness that each woman journeys through when faced with challenges of disorders of the reproductive organs, whether it is endometriosis, infertility, polycystic ovaries, or another. Certainly, the journey seems dark and hopeless and in this despair we are willing to leave what we know, because in this place we really do not know the answer to WHY. And out of desperation, only when faced with these circumstances, are we willing to explore and open ourselves to search deeply, whole heartedly as if our life depended on it, because from our limited perspective our life does depend on it. It becomes the forefront of our daily living, a persistent annoyance that grows each day seeking only complete resolution within our whole being.

It is my hope and intention that this book can serve as a guiding light to help you unravel the entanglement and walk through the maze of discoveries within your being in hopes that it will lead you to experience greater truth of the treasure that you are. With sincerity and persistence you may even discover that what seemed to be a curse turns out to be a real blessing in disguise. And it is my hope and intention that you discover that jewel, to be able to live in the peace, joy and beauty that is our divine fulfillment. This jewel within is the true essence of what the true Feminine is all about.

Perhaps this jewel is the light at the end of the tunnel, the discovery of yourself unveiled in the Truth. The journey of this book is to assist you in your walking to this deeper side within yourself, where you can allow yourself to embrace the beauty, love, peace, joy and happiness of wholeness that exists inside. This is the journey of discovering our own true jewel and allowing this wholeness to permeate throughout our being, which essentially heals us emotionally, mentally and also physically. We all carry this jewel; there are no exceptions to this rule.

Wholeness is available for each and every one of us, but it is our responsibility to choose it, to turn within, let go of our pain and suffering and open up to a greater reality of ourselves. In order to achieve and live in the reality of wholeness we have to let go of what doesn't work for us, let go of who we thought we were and step into who we really are.

This book first focuses on a conversation of what healing and wholeness is, with the intention of allowing your minds to grasp and taste the possibilities available. Secondly, we'll continue to explore various aspect of our being in order to heal our physical body, while unraveling some of our limiting beliefs, thoughts, emotions and old patterns that interfere with our state of health and wellness. As we continue, walking through the mental, emotional, and physical aspects of healing, we'll then conclude with a chapter on Spirituality, which truly permeates through the subtle levels of consciousness.

It is helpful to read one chapter at a time and take the time to practice and incorporate some of the changes that you discover as you advance along the book. Use the book as a tool, not just as information. Try to incorporate the practices that will allow you to feel good and embrace greater wholeness and healing.
Enjoy your journey towards yourself, best of wishes!!!

CONTENTS

CHAPTER 1

Most Asked Question: Why Me?

Mostly, every woman that I have ever treated has asked the question of "Why Me?" Why am I experiencing infertility, endometriosis or cancer? What does it mean? Why is this happening to me?

It is the question we ask to try to make sense of our situation. The conventional medical community of experts can answer that question with the physical interactions that take place and can explain the condition from the view of its physiology. They can explain the disease in its relationship with the physical body and its disease state. But many times the answer to why you are experiencing this disease or disorder is much more complicated than that and really may have many answers on many levels. There is probably a corresponding answer on the mental, emotional, physical and spiritual levels of consciousness as well. I suspect that most people take home with them the physical explanation and even though they are not completely satisfied, they accept that as the complete truth and settle for that answer. Many others begin their search into these others levels of consciousness and try literally to make sense and understand the physical disorder from a much deeper, profound way.

The question of "Why Me?" becomes louder and harder to deny when there is no physical explanation for your diagnosis. For example, in the case of unexplained Infertility, medical doctors may find no apparent reason for the fact that the couple is not able to conceive. It appears allusive and mysterious and harder to accept in our mind. Somehow it is easier to accept a medical condition that has reasoning behind it as its explanation, rather than no apparent medical reason at all. It is easier to accept because then the disorder is justified on the physical level; in other words there now is a reason, and we can leave it at that, if we choose to or we can follow our instincts and dive deeper into our psyche to find out what else could be causing these conditions in our body.

Physiological answers for gynecological and fertility related issues are easy to find as well as other contributing factors such as nutritional deficiencies, stress issues, lack of exercise, overwork, etc.. Yet none of these answers really suffice what these affected women want to know in their hearts, "Why Me?" And clearly many times failure to conceive and gynecological disorders are definitely linked to stress factors, daily habits and behaviors, as well as lifestyle and nutritional health. Yet correcting these factors does not guarantee correcting the problem. So when you have corrected all the daily stress factors and bad habits and diet, what then is the answer to the most asked question in Women's diagnosis: "Why Me?

Perhaps the answer lies within. Let's take a look at what wholeness is and how it may relate to the question of "Why?"

What Is Wholeness?

Wholeness is the true state of our nature within. As we experience life, we can either identify who we are with a concept of limitation, fear and lack, or we can see through these illusions of our ego and acknowledge the wholeness within. In those terms, wholeness is the acknowledgement that we are whole to begin with. That our being is whole and that even though we usually experience the parts of the pie rather than the pie completely, we acknowledge that we are much more than our current experience at each moment.

Wholeness means that we are not lacking in anything, regardless of what our limited experience is. Therefore we already possess the peace, love and joy, as well as many of the other qualities that we are constantly seeking for outside ourselves. Are feelings of fear, anger, and sadness are not who we really are, we just experience these feelings. At our core, we are the whole that experiences the emotions, the thoughts, the images and we are the things that we experience. We are a spirit having a human experience. And as a spirit or soul, we are whole and able to embrace variations of emotional and mental states.

Having wholeness means that our being is designed in the image of the oneness, the vital source and vital energy. Our body has the innate ability to return and restore itself to wholeness and health when the body finds itself out of balance. This is true for mostly all parts of ourselves. The design of wholeness is at the core of our being. We are made in the perfect image of the divine, meaning that the treasure is buried within us. We have inherent in our being (soul) the ability to heal our body, our hearts, our mind and our emotions. Our being is whole and able to connect with that truth within us, which is a level of consciousness existing deep in our hearts. To be connected and aware of this consciousness allows us the freedom from our other limiting patterns of consciousness that creates disease in the human body.

By connecting to our wholeness, we can experience a place deep within ourselves that feels whole and good, without needing anything from outside to fill our needs. In this place, we can experience our Self as an essence of love and we can be at peace with the world outside ourselves, as well as within ourselves.

To feel our wholeness means to feel the part of ourselves that is also known as our spiritual essence. In that place we are whole. There is no need, there is no pain, there is no lack, and there is no imbalance or disharmony.

This state of wholeness is possible to embrace, but what happens is that our mental and emotional patterns limit us and block us from experiencing our complete truth of wholeness within. In other words, our "ego" has created an illusion of separation from our true essence and source, and then functions on these patterns of limiting beliefs, as if they were completely true.

From a psychological standpoint, in our everyday experience, we have created beliefs that we will call pictures; around lack (feeling like we are not enough, or there is not enough in the world), limitation, and fear. Even though these beliefs/pictures are not complete truths, we still completely submit to them because it is the reality from which we function day to day and what is familiar to us.

In other words, if we experience any physical disorder, our first response is immediately to default to a feeling of not good enough or unworthiness because this situation is happening to us. This is based on a buried belief that we unconsciously took on at some point in our lives and now we use our outer circumstances to

7

reinforce and support our limiting picture of ourselves. The truth is we are whole, and our event of experiencing any disease state does not define us as being "good" or "not", but in our mental and emotionally consciousness we experience it that way. These are the pictures we create that interfere with our health and wellbeing.

The truth is that these beliefs and pictures have been there all along for many, many generations. As we evolve and move towards greater levels of consciousness, it is only natural for us to move towards our wholeness and evolve all the aspects of our emotional and mental consciousness. These situations outside of ourselves are only opportunities to bring these places of limitation to awareness and help us evolve them by dispelling the old beliefs. These situations, concerning our health, trigger our places of pain and suffering and force us to look at what we really are believing and living in our lives. Ultimately, if we choose, it becomes an opportunity to connect and free ourselves from the pain and suffering in our mental and emotional levels of consciousness and bring light and healing to our physical body.

How Exactly Does This Help Me Heal My Physical Condition?

You may be wondering how exactly does this heal your body. Here is the answer: It will help you bring health to your physical body; whether it's conceiving, healing endometriosis, or any other physical or emotional disorder by exploring the underlying emotional, mental and spiritual aspects that are contributing to your physical disorder.

As we experience more and more limiting levels of consciousness as thought forms and emotions, our bodies are affected by their own ability to function at the level of health within. Our bodies start shutting down and functioning from that place of lack and limitation, which limits the oxygen, creates stress, and alters the biochemistry to our detriment. This in turn creates disease and dysfunction in our bodies.

Our thought patterns, and emotional states as well as our spiritual alignment all contribute to our physical health. When we are holding thoughts of fear, lack and limitation, unconsciously we create blockages in the body, which affect the overall energy and functioning of the organ systems. Once the organ systems are affected we see and experience disease and disorders.

Let's think of our wholeness consciousness as being a white light that continuously feeds every aspect of our human physical body with all the precise medicine and nutrients that it needs to stay functioning perfectly. Then, comes a layer of emotions that are holding fears, doubts and shameful feelings which we have enslaved ourselves to unconsciously. These feelings are dense and block the light from reaching certain aspects of our physical body; as if the sun can not reach a plant. That plant is our physical body not getting the correct "light" it needs to function properly, grow and sustain itself.

Consequently, over that layer we add another layer of mental distress of all the limiting thoughts we have incorporated into our consciousness, in which we have defined our very existence with. This further dims our light and creates more barriers, blocking that essential life giving light from reaching places in our physical bodies. So, in the end we are left with a physical body that is disconnected from our core essence and disconnected from the life-giving energy that is needed for our bodies to function optimally. Like a plant without any sunlight we can't expect to be healthy and vibrant.

In conclusion, we each hold various emotions, thoughts and beliefs in our body/mind/ and psyche. These beliefs/pictures and emotions create blockages that can create disease and disorders in the physical body, thus interfering with our body's ability to be healthy and function optimally. These aspects all contribute to our overall health and wellbeing, not just of the reproductive system.

For example, many unexplained infertility patients worry and become fearful every month about not becoming pregnant. In turn, the constant worrying will affect the spleen and kidney organ system, as well as others, which can create stagnation and deficiency, depleting the body further and making fertility more and more real. Therefore, it becomes a viscous cycle where the physical symptoms (unexplained infertility), impacts the mental aspect (thinking it will never happen), further impacts the emotional state (feeling worried and fearful) and creates further tensions and stress, which alters the biochemistry of the body and does not let the body function optimally. These continued patterns deteriorate the body further, creating more disease, pain and suffering and more of those limiting layers of pictures.

Throughout this book, our journey will be to experience various ways in which we can transform some of these limiting layers of pictures that are interfering with our body's ability to stay healthy or create health, especially in the reproductive area.

In essence, what we are doing is finding ways to heal our physical body, specifically our reproductive area by connecting with our core wholeness consciousness of our soul. Staying in alignment with this wholeness consciousness not only allows us to heal our bodies physically, but also allows us to feel more joy and love and less pain and suffering in our lives and bodies.

Wholistic Medicine then in turn, is the medicine that we use when we are addressing the wholeness of who we are. It is very similar to Alternative Medicine but the main difference is the direction it is meant to take you. Where Alternative Medicine is a catch all for medicine that is not "conventional or allopathic", Wholistic medicine strives to connect us to the wholeness consciousness of our soul. There is an inherent belief with Wholistic Medicine that our bodies are whole even though we have separated ourselves from this wholeness, and it is our journey to become fully aware of this reality (consciousness) of wholeness in order to restore our physical, emotional, mental and spiritual health.

Getting Started

In the clinical setting I use various forms of alternative medicine; Traditional Chinese Medicine, Acupuncture, Chinese Herbology, Nutrition, Emotional Coaching, Spiritual Healing and counseling in order to assist in the process of healing and restoring health in the body. Then our work begins and evolves with each session as the body integrates the changes and moves forward.

Most sessions include a combination of the in order to help patients reach the truth of who they are and open up to the healing that that brings. Some sessions include more talk about nutrition and what is happening in someone's body in relationship to that, while other sessions may include more healing and spiritual work.

All in all, our sessions include a comprehensive evaluation, with a personalized detail attention to what each person may need to continue to heal and move forward in her life.

While it may be important to work with a professional for life changing opportunities, it is really the changes that are maintained on a daily basis that make the difference in your life. This type of healing medicine includes participation on behalf of the patient, it is not about coming in and receiving a treatment and walking away. Things change in a treatment and therefore you change, your views may change, your attitudes change, your beliefs change, your life changes, so therefore your health changes. I often tell patients, when they come in for the first time, that it is about them, it is up to them how much they really want to receive from coming here, not about the treatments.

From that perspective, it is important for patients to incorporate daily practices that will cultivate and support these changes and shifts in their consciousness, such as meditation, journaling, aromatherapy points, and other spiritual practices. Many of the following tools are just for that, to create awareness and facilitate the healing process in each one of you. These tools will not necessarily replace treatments but it can enhance your choice of treatments and make changes in your lives that will create real change.

I present to you in the following chapters an intricate understanding of how our body's health is affected by the more subtle aspect of our being; our mind, emotions and spiritual bodies. Along with this understanding we include practices that I have been successfully employing for quite a few years in our treatments of fertility. It is my belief that using this book as a reference and a guidebook, may lead to healing these subtle layers that we mentioned in our being. It may be necessary to also add some alternative medicine to your healing process, or receive some Emotional coaching along the way, but the most important thing is that the work is really up to you and you have most of the tools right here in this book to facilitate your own healing.

However, it is important to acknowledge that using this book or any other form of Alternative Medicine is not a substitute for having a responsible western medical workup and diagnosis, if you are experiencing a physical disease or disorder. It is important to have all the proper lab work and diagnosis work completed and then you may decide what the best treatment course is for you.

Embarking on this road may change your body, as well as your life. So, enjoy the journey.

CHAPTER 2

Nourishing the Transformation of Change

Patient Case Histories

Patient Case Hillary: Chronic Miscarriage and Unexplained Infertility

Hillary was a wonderful 34 year old that wanted to get pregnant. She had had miscarriages in the past and came in to be helped with both issues, fertility and miscarriages. Patient Hillary became pregnant very quickly after about five weeks of receiving Acupuncture and Chinese Medicine treatments. One day she came in, about five weeks pregnant and stated she felt great but had some apprehension about her miscarriage pattern. She didn't seem to want to really acknowledge any of the feelings of doubt and fear concerning the possibility of miscarriages occurring again, understandably so. Here she was, five weeks pregnant (undoubtedly what she had been hoping for), yet she said, "I am just counting the days to get past this time…I just can't bare this time of waiting until I am in a much more secure place." This being an all too familiar statement, amongst my patients, I looked over and felt into what she was saying.

As I glanced over at her, I could perceive a shadow and heaviness over the left side of her heart. This is where she was holding pain, isolated from the rest of her heart, where she was feeling comfortable. I gently brought her awareness to this place of pain and she could see how much she was avoiding this place because it felt wrong to her to have feelings that were so negative and scary, as if confronting this place within herself could make her worst fears come true. She was concerned that if she felt these negative feelings then somehow she would bring on her own negative result. If she felt her fear about losing the pregnancy then she would actually bring on the miscarriage.

She also did not want to look at these feelings within herself because she had an expectation of herself to be "strong" and "not wallow in her misery". She felt that feeling these feelings somehow felt "weak" and "she should know better." All these statements were common amongst my patients and many who continuously confuse being strong with having very little emotional fluctuations or have any emotions at all. So, in turn we suppress these emotions and do not allow them to have an outlet.

In my experience, I have learned that it is the very fact of suppressing these emotions, rather than experiencing them, that cause disruption in our physical body. When we suppress emotions by not giving them an outlet, they create disruption and blockage of that light that gives us the essence of life itself that we discussed in the analogy before. This blockage leads to disorders and patterns of disease. It disrupts the patterns of life and health that are innate in our physical body.

Hillary realized how she was pushing aside this area of pain in herself and how she did not want to look at it or acknowledge it because of her fears and misconceptions. But now she was looking at it and noticing that this place was there in her heart. And that she could just allow this place in her heart to be there, surrounded by love and compassion from a higher source and accept it for what it was. As she did this, she could feel some of those feelings of grief, sadness and despair from her past experiences. She realized she could just be open to giving herself permission to feel the grief of those past moments in her life, without carrying over the identification of that experience into the present scenario. In other words, by confronting this picture of pain from her past, she was able to let it go and not continue to subconsciously fear that it would happen again. She was able to just be with those feelings, not having to fix anything or change it, or make the time go faster, or deny them in any way.

As she allowed herself the courage to look at this place within herself; she said, "It takes a lot of energy just to keep myself from looking at this place within me and trying to be perfect or good enough". She realized in that moment that she was good enough, and that before she had identified with not being good enough because of her experience of having lost her babies. Through blaming and shaming herself, she had attributed the loss of her babies to how good she was or wasn't, to her self worth. By looking at this pattern directly for what it was, she was able to reconnect with her true essence; her wholeness consciousness and realize it was just a layer of emotions and thoughts that were not necessarily true, but that she believed as true.

The truth is that we are good enough. For Hillary, being "good enough" meant not having any of those feelings that were considered "negative." What she realized in those few minutes was that having these feelings did not mean she wasn't good enough, it was her "belief or pictures" about them that were telling her she wasn't good enough when she had these feelings. At that level of consciousness, Patient H was never going to feel good enough because it is impossible to be completely free of "negative feelings" or unpleasant emotions. It is part of our humanity to have feelings such as fear, grief, sadness, despair, etc… that do not feel good. Now, by feeling that she is good enough and that she also has these feelings, changes her whole outlook of herself and will have astounding effects on her wellbeing and her health. Now she is that much more connected to her truth, her wholeness consciousness and that light shines through dispelling the pictures that were causing physical imbalance. This may very well be enough life force released to assist her in carrying a pregnancy full term.

And indeed it was, her baby girl was born healthy and well nine months later. As we look at the dynamics of Hillary, we see that understandably so, she hadn't allowed herself to integrate the part of herself that felt the heaviness of the past miscarriages and the grief around that. This was too much for her to bear without having a way to fix it. Why would she voluntarily open herself up to these feelings without a way to fix them? And if she had a way to fix them she would have "gotten rid of these long time ago." So she was feeling cornered with no way out, which is a common feeling among patients. This pain stayed frozen in time- weighing heavily on her, without an apparent way out. This pain had been there for a while and it wasn't new but now it was triggered by her recurrence of pregnancy against a background of miscarriages (her feared prognosis).

The misconception Hillary had was that we cannot express our negative feelings otherwise we will bring on a negative outcome, which really corners us into staying stuck in a holding patterns with our pain. We feel trapped in not being able to express any emotions unless they are pleasant or otherwise "positive", such as t happiness, joy, and love. This is very limiting and we would all be robots if we would walk around like this. As part of being human, we experience fear, grief, sadness, anger, rage, and many, many other emotions. It is the fact of actually experiencing these emotions and dispelling their hold on us, that leads to health in our bodies. There is a difference between acknowledging and experiencing our emotions versus living in a constant level of negativity. We fall in to negativity when we feel our negative emotions and then believe that that reality is the only reality. When we can not see beyond our limiting patterns to the truth that lies underneath the feelings of despair and pain, we feel trapped.

The place of "I am not good enough" is a very common picture within all of our consciousness, especially as a woman in our society. This is a common pattern for many patients. And it is a pattern that is evident in the fabric of our society and yet very hidden. Addressing this picture within your consciousness, as it may surface throughout your fertility treatments, may very well be the key to creating more health in your physical body. These and other similar pictures come up as you become aware of what you are feeling and believing. Then we can just face these places, and allow the essence in our breath to disintegrate these pictures. This is the moment of choice, where we come to choose if we want to keep believing and living from that limited belief and picture or if we want to trust a higher source or vibration, which is operating within us and around us. We get to choose, and our choice will determine our health and our healing. And the beauty is we don't have to fix it, just bring these pictures to the higher source of life; the light of the divine within us. By holding it in compassion and love, it amazingly integrates into the highest place, if we choose.

Patient Alexandra- Infertility, Stage 1 endometriosis and three failed IVF's

Alexandra was a vibrant beautiful young woman in her early 30s who exuded beauty, softness and excitement. She came in to see me for a few sessions because she had had a couple of failed IVFs and wanted to try again and do everything in her power to improve her condition. As she worked with me we journeyed into a place of pain and suffering that she held in her belly. Although she was scared that her IVF would fail again, she decided to go ahead with it. I could tell that she was in a lot of turmoil about it. As she moved deeper into her heart, she realized she was in pain and also jealous of her friend's new baby. Over her jealousy of her friend's baby, she was angry at herself for even daring to feel jealousy, which made her feel more shameful about herself.

As we moved through the anger she accepted the jealousy,

Alexandra felt her deep shame, shame that told her she was wrong. She was wrong for feeling jealousy, wrong for everything in her life, she felt like a complete failure. And when she tuned into her body she could feel this wrongness as pressure in her ovaries and in her whole pelvic area.

Alexandra realized that she had been feeling wrong due to her personal history and her past; Her step father would continuously tell her how wrong she was always and her mother criticized her all her life. She was also hurt by her father's abandonment and her brother's rejection of her. She had interpreted all these events as being a failure in someway. And further more, she interpreted the reason she was wrong was because she was a female. Perhaps if she would have been a male, her life would have been different, she thought, and perhaps others would have loved her and accepted her in a different way. So unconsciously, being female was part of her failure, so that energy of being wrong was held in the deepest part of herself, her female organs.

Once she became in touch with the belief and pictures these thought patterns generated, then she came to a place of choice. And she could then choose to continue believing this or turn to a higher source within and listening to the truth of her being and her self worth.

In our session, Alexandra was able to move deeper into her heart and feel her true essence, the Divine essence that has nothing to do with other people's reaction to her. Her essence was untouched and she could now start to bring her consciousness into that reality of who she really was. She was a beautiful, loving, caring, and a strong women that wasn't wrong for being alive or being born. She could see beyond the negative voice of not having a right to exist. She could see that she had the right, as much as everyone else and that right was from the highest source. There were no mistakes about her existence and her worthiness; it had just been her limited interpretation all along.

As with Alexandra, many women, live with the unconscious belief that they are not worthy, because of the conditional love that they received when they were little and because of the limited interpretation of the events in their past. When women make themselves feel wrong about our femaleness, their bodies hold all that distortion in their female organs and of course, that affects their physiological bio-chemistry.

In conclusion, Alexandra had a beautiful baby boy with her next attempt at IVF, assisted with wholistic medicine; traditional Chinese medicine and healing sessions and emotional Coaching.

Patient Veronica – Endometriosis and Infertility

Patient Veronica came in to my office with a long history of endometriosis. As we began the sessions she told me how she felt. "As a woman", I feel like it has always been a very hard thing. I got my period when I was 9 years old. I was traumatized. No one told me what to do. Then I always had pain with my periods and there were so many things I couldn't do, I wasn't like my brothers, they had all the freedom. Then, I had such bad luck in relationships and then I got breast cancer, and now I may have the ovarian cancer gene."

I could clearly see the pain that Veronica was in and how she saw her female body as something that caused her so much pain rather than joy, something negative. She could feel the pain increase in her ovaries and lower back as she spoke these words. She believed that she was doomed basically because she was a woman. She could feel the heaviness of her thoughts, especially of her thought that being a woman meant all those negative things. She had, in many ways identified herself as a woman with pain and suffering, and the most interesting thing was that her body responded with more pain when she spoke about it.

During our session, Veronica was able to see that perhaps her negative thoughts and blaming herself about her womanhood was the root cause of her pain and suffering and perhaps there was an undiscovered truth underneath the heaviness of all the pain and suffering. As she delved into her pain and allowed herself to be filled with the essence in her breath and perhaps surrendering to something bigger than herself, she started to feel lighter and more peaceful.

As she asked the divine light that was coming in with each breath, what the truth of her being really was, she started to feel less pain in these areas of pain in her ovaries and her lower back; she started to feel lighter, happier and more peaceful.

Veronica started to feel different in her body, the heaviness and ache in all other places had disappeared and she started to experience herself differently than before. She could feel herself full of light and love, and she could see that there was a whole other dimension for her to explore about herself that she hadn't even entered until now. All this pain in her body had brought her to a new place as she faced the limitations of her own belief.

Even though Veronica still had a journey of discovery in front of her, she was now able to move into new terrain. She was no longer stuck in the old mind frame of pain and suffering, as she had lived for so many years. She was willing to let go of her old thoughts about her womanhood. Her physical body was now a little freer from the constraints of her old belief patterns and did not need to continue to create disease and destruction in order to stay in congruency with her beliefs about herself. She was freer to experience the truth about who she really was and begin to function, instead, from that place of peace, harmony and beauty within her.

Throughout our sessions, Veronica healed her body and her emotions and went on to have a beautiful baby girl. She healed her endometriosis. Furthermore, she felt completely different about herself and could now pass that on to a new generation.

How We Abandon Ourselves

For women and sometimes men, there is a pattern, which I will demonstrate in the next case story, in which we keep sacrificing ourselves to try to find happiness. The pattern is something like this: If we deny ourselves of our true feelings, abandoning our own self, in the attempt to avoid conflict or a difference of opinion with another person, then we think we will make the other person happy, in turn making ourselves happy because the other person will not leave and stay to love us.

In other words, we do not allow ourselves to say what we are feeling to another in order to maintain the peace and receive the love; we completely abandon ourselves and end up playing a game that leaves us feeling empty and disappointed.

The love we receive isn't really clean, but yet we have the manipulated outcome that we thought will give us the love and peace that we all deeply seek. Then we are left with these unspoken feelings within our self of what we really wanted to say, but didn't, because of fear of abandonment; and yet we ended up abandoning ourselves. Where did all those feelings go? They have to be hidden somewhere. We hide them deep, deep inside ourselves, and many times as women, in our reproductive system.

Does this pattern really keep the peace? No, it doesn't, because it is impossible for us to have peace when we have abandoned our true feelings, and are hiding out of fear. The fear has pervaded over authenticity of our expression and there is a price to pay.

What is the price? The price is usually your body, your health, your womanhood, your peace. We give up the very thing that we are looking for.

Patient: Claudia – Unexplained Infertility, 1 failed IVF
Claudia came in and said that she was frustrated at her husband

29

because they had had a fight the night before. "But now" she said, everything is okay and I was able to fix it with a phone call."

I asked her, how did she do that?

"Well, I just called him and said that I was wrong and that I loved him very much." She replied.

"Oh I see", I said, then I asking, "How did that feel to you?"

"It feels sad and disappointing" she said. "And I am frustrated that I always have to be the one to call him up and say that or else he storms out."

This went on for a while during our session, until Claudia noticed that we had moved into her sadness. She felt that her sadness was about feeling like he had betrayed her, and continued to betray her in the relationship because his focus was always himself. She felt trapped and abandoned.

Then I asked her, "Do you see what is happening, who has really abandoned you?" "Myself," she answered. "Because I feel that if I say what I want to say then he leaves, I have to be what he wants me to be so that I can have his love. But the truth is I feel frustrated and angry that he is selfish and that I cannot be me."

On a deep level Claudia has attached herself to the belief that she is unlovable and that the only way for her to feel the love from this man is to make him feel like he is right and she is wrong, then he will stay and she will be happy to have someone that loves her. The truth is that she is not happy, she is deeply upset, frustrated and feels alone and abandoned in this relationship. She is not feeling loved even though she is doing all that she thinks she needs to do in order for herself to feel the love.

As we continued to work, her emotional pain of her relationship was felt by her in her ovaries. When she felt the pain and sadness in her heart, she could feel the physical pain in her ovaries. This showed us both a direct correlation to where she was holding her pain in her body.

On a deeper level, in that same session, Claudia realized that she was really abandoning her self by not allowing her truth to be expressed. She was taking responsibility over all his doings and making herself feel wrong in the relationship. This was her deep wound of feeling wrong in life and it was playing out in her relationship with her husband. This feeling of being wrong and unworthy of love was also playing out in her ovaries and reproductive system, affecting her ability to conceive.

As we moved through layers of pain, Claudia unveiled the truth. She was able to see that she really wasn't unworthy of love, or defective in her core. She was a beautiful design made by the highest light of Divine source. And just like everyone else, she was deserving of love. She did not have to play this game of making herself feel wrong to receive the love. She could feel the love and peace, directly from the source inside herself and yes through others. She realized in her rational mind that yes, this was her husband, but ultimately not the source of the love, only the divine is the source of the love, and that was already well established in her, she just had to open herself to this knowing inside herself.

Two months later Claudia conceived and then nine months later delivered a beautiful baby girl.

Above, in Claudia's case you have the old limiting belief pattern vs. the truth of who we are manifesting in our body physically in the ovaries. It is no surprise that this belief would manifest in her ovaries, due to the fact that it is about her own belief of who she is as a woman. A woman is defined in many ways including through our reproductive organs.

These two places within her may continue to play out, until she is well established in her knowing about her own truth. She may play out this a few more times in her relationship, but perhaps may stop herself and have a more honest conversation with her husband the following time. Instead of dishonestly taking responsibility in order to avoid a difference of opinion, she may risk saying, "I love you very much, and I know that usually say that I was wrong, but if I do that I would not be dishonest with you. What I feel is that I have a different opinion than you and that doesn't make either one of us wrong; can we dialogue about this?" This would leave an array of possibilities to be discussed, rather than a win or lose situation, wrong or right, good or bad.

Furthermore, this type of honest communication about what she is feeling allows her to take care of herself, not abandon herself and not feel betrayed by herself nor by him for having a different opinion. And even more importantly, it doesn't need for her to store her hidden feelings somewhere else, and therefore her body is able to begin the healing process and restore the integrity of the system.

Walking Toward Wholeness

As we read all of the above cases, we start to look and understand how the levels of consciousness affect our physical body in a very real way. Now while everyone is different, of course, and while all women share on some level some insecurity of our bodies and of our species, we do not always have gynecological or fertility related disorders. Yes this is true. But for some of us it does manifest in our reproductive system. Instead of asking why, I just prefer to accept its manifestation wherever it may be and let the underlying causes behind it unravel.

Maybe for other women our feminine pain body (as Eckart Tolle would say) may manifest as weight issues, or in those that have a deep desire to have extensive plastic surgery to alter their physical body. It is apparent in our society that being a woman is something that we are continuing to define and continuing to search for peace, individually and in the mass consciousness. While some women are completely at peace with their femininity and who they are on all levels, most of us continue to work through it and towards the discovery of our wholeness.

All the patients above were able to connect to their mental pictures and beliefs, the emotional pain derived from those and deeper aspect of their being that were contributing to the manifestation of their current limiting physical state of infertility. In the process, they discovered deep spiritual truths about themselves that freed them from these limiting states of consciousness. By acquiring this freer state of mind, emotion and spirit, they freed their physical body from the restriction of the disorder and restored their innate state of health. Their bodies then continued the natural process of conceiving because it is the natural order of life. They had no other obstacles in the way.

By beginning exactly where you are, with what you are experiencing and moving through each layer, freeing you mental, emotional and spiritual body, you automatically move into wholeness. Wholeness is not a state to achieve out there, it is already a state of consciousness that exists within you and all you have to do is to be willing to let go of the pictures, beliefs and accompanying emotions that do not let you experience that truth.

The following chapters and pages are designed with that intention in mind. They are designed to help you walk towards wholeness consciousness and embrace that reality within yourself and all of humankind.

CHAPTER 3

Transforming our Mental Body

How Our Thoughts Affect Our Body

In the previous chapter we discussed the basis of wholism and of a True self. We believe essentially that the journey to your True self is full of all possibilities and has the ability to heal and create health within our bodies. This is what we are calling our True Self. This is our divine aspect of ourself, which we can project from the world outside ourselves. This True Self is therefore the highest vibration of our being. This is important to keep in mind, when we start to talk about our belief system and how to raise the vibrations of our thoughts to create health within.

The mind is a powerful aspect of ourselves. All our thoughts and perceptions, actively affect our physical biochemistry. In other words each thought corresponds to a bio chemical in our body. Every thought we have may produce an emotion, a feeling and an experience in our body. When we think of something scary, for example, or perceive something to be scary, we may feel the fear as an emotion and then feel a physical tightening of our stomach. This physical reaction correlates to biochemical changes that take place simultaneously within our perception. In other words, the moment we perceive something, our brain releases signals in form of chemical reactions and causes changes all throughout the body, thus we experience the tightness in our stomachs. Because of these bio-chemical reactions, our glandular systems are affected as well, and in turn affect our reproductive system completely.

When we have unconscious judgments, self doubt or other self defeating pictures or beliefs about ourselves, we begin to give the physical body a mixed message. This mixed message defeats every effort of healing our fertility and reproductive imbalances because our physiology is a reflection of our mental, emotional, and spiritual states. Our subconscious beliefs are held deeply which simultaneously act with our physical body and bio-chemistry. Therefore, until these beliefs or pictures are released consciously or brought to awareness, they continue to contribute to your physical state of health or lack of health. Our body is constantly communicating with us through a series of chemical reactions, signs and symptoms. And our mental thoughts are very influential in creating the physical states of health that we experience.

For example, we may have a belief that says "This will never work, I will never get pregnant", underlining all your efforts. There may be partial truth to this if your age is reflective of 40 or older; nonetheless, there is a great amount of entangled fear and hopelessness underlining that statement. Other unconscious belief or voices could be, "I am not getting pregnant because I probably do not deserve it", or "things never go right for me, and this will not work out either". These underlining voices that are unconscious drive your body's chemistry and continue to support this negative statement in your being until that thought is made conscious, or you become aware that that thought is operating in you. Knowing this, you could understand why it may be so overwhelmingly difficult to conceive, even when medical doctors cannot find anything wrong with you.

Reproductive disorders can be a reflection of many underlining pictures and beliefs; our worthiness to create, worthiness to bring forth some level of creation, self judgments and doubts of our womanhood, our bodies, our relationships, our intimacy with our partners, etc. Through self analysis we may discover what these underlining pictures and beliefs are and allowing these places within us to heal. As we continue this journey with great compassion for ourselves, we can gently dive into these sensitive places and bring light and allow our true shining light to come forth in health and healing.

So, in lieu of that, let us continue the journey of opening ourselves up to becoming aware of our unconscious mental attitudes and releasing them so that they do not continue to unconsciously govern our health and our body.

Setting Your Mind for Healing

Let us begin with a set of principles that will help you sail through this journey with much more ease. These next few items of this list will set up a state of mind for you that will assist you in healing your body. Please read thoroughly and try to open yourself up to perceiving things from the following perspective. It will aid in releasing limiting conditioning pictures and beliefs.

Be Willing to Stay Open Minded

Staying open minded allows you to let other possibilities come in to your life, by the pure law of attraction. If we stay closed believing that things will not work, that there are no options; then we don't even allow the possibility of options to come our way. By adopting an open mental attitude you can explore various avenues and consider options that are non-traditional. You also give yourself a chance to open up to all possibilities rather than thinking that you have reached the end of the road.

Allow yourself to open your mind and emotions to all possibilities. Making assumptions and conclusions prematurely closes your options. Seek many opinions, until you hear the answer that resonates in your heart, rather than in your head. Sometimes that answer may be to take a break, to resolve relationship issues, or to continue with treatment. Always check the thoughts against your heart and feel what is right for you.

Be Willing To Learn Something New About Your Body

Many times we think we have heard it all and yet there is a whole world inside of ourselves that will amaze us. Our physical issues are much more than what is represented in the surface. Please give yourself the opportunity to discover the beauty within.

Acknowledge That You Have a Vital Energy And Be Willing To Trust It

Start to become aware of the deep inner source that is really directing the show. This represents your vital energy and is at the core of your wellbeing. Trusting this helps you gain perspective into your personal situation more easily. Whether you call it a vital force, God, ALLAH, Divine Light, ALLAHA, Divine Love, etc... it is all the same vital force of goodness and healing.

Be Willing To Believe That Physical Change Is Possible

As we mentioned in the previous chapter, the concept of being more than you see is a very important piece in creating health in your body. Allow yourself to believe that you are much more than meets the eye. Exploring each aspect of your being with the understanding that it all contributes to health, as well as to disease, gives you great freedom in receiving healing.

Be Willing to Push Yourself Beyond Your Comfort Level

When we are exploring new avenues, we may not be as comfortable or familiar as we normally are. Other friends or family members may not be as encouraging only because it is not familiar territory. Be willing to investigate and push your limits on what you used to think and what may be your new thinking now, expand your horizon.

Be Willing To Dedicate 100% to Yourself

Be willing to give yourself time and treat yourself to new things. Getting off the track of everyday "have to and should's" SHOULD be on your list of things to do. It is important to change what you have been doing so that you get different results than what you have been getting. Pay attention to your needs they are very, very important.

Be Willing To Honor Yourself, Your Feelings, Your Journey

Honor yourself, your process, your feelings, even if it is different than anyone else's. Just because it is different than someone else's doesn't mean that you are worse than them, or better than them. It doesn't mean anything about you; it only shows you that you are engaged in a process and are identifying yourself with that thought. Do not identify your self worth with your physical circumstances or condition, in other words, if you find yourself facing difficulty, that does not mean there is something wrong with you. The circumstances do not determine your worth. Getting hung up on the meanings or interpreting the process distracts you from and can be damaging to the healing process.

We honor ourselves by also honoring our needs. What is it that we need in this moment to move forward with healing? Do we need to relax, take a break, make a decision, not make a decision? What do we need right now in this moment, knowing that tomorrow you may access again your needs and make a different decision? The decision you make is just for now, the moment at hand. Honor our needs with compassion, not judgement for having those needs. We deserve the compassion and understanding from ourselves to begin with. While honoring our needs, it is important to also accept that situation and condition for what it is, rather than desperately trying

43

to change it. When we are able to be in a place of acceptance with our physical condition, then we can allow whatever changes need to occur much easier and without resistance. Acceptance is an important key to our healing.

Be Willing To Take Responsibility for What Isn't Working

Sometimes when things aren't working we think we are automatically doomed and we spiral down into a field of negativity and damaging thoughts about ourselves and who we are. Become aware that when something doesn't work according to plan, it is not a definition of who you are in any way. It doesn't mean you are wrong, bad or unworthy in any way.

Secondly, recognize that you have options, and sometimes the options may look dim, but many times they offer a gift in disguise. Sometimes, in order for us to explore another road we may have to be forced into a different path than expected, and what we knew may no longer be an option. There is an old saying; "one door may have to close in order for another door to open". Remember that saying when things look hopeless and know that you may just be in between doors.

Meet Disappointment with Curiosity

When we acknowledge that there is a deeper connection guiding the pace of our lives, then it becomes easier to trust that there is order in our lives. Many times we may not get what we think we want, or perhaps maybe not when we think we need it or through the avenue that we want, and yet there is a higher order in place, a door waiting to be opened.

Meeting disappointment with an openness of exploring that door helps us move closer to our healing, rather than sink into suffering and negative pictures about what we think our disappointment means. Each step becomes a process of a new discovery by inviting curiosity. Allow it to be just that; by staying open if things do not turn out as expected and seeing where the next piece leads you. Stay curious as to what you may discover within yourself and what treasures it may bring.

Be Willing To Be In the "Not Knowing"

I find that an obstacle that stops patients from seeking healing for their female conditions is the "not knowing" phase. This is when the ability a woman has of solving the problem is not readily available in her mind and she automatically presumes that she had to succumb to the problem and that there is no solution because she cannot "figure it out."

45

In other words, a patient may have been diagnosed with unexplained infertility and after a few failed IVF's (In Vitro-Fertilizations) the patient decides that her system is not working so she will give up, because on the surface it seems that there is no answer to her dilemma. The patient is in a space of not knowing. And because the space of not knowing is a difficult one to be in because of previous conditioning, shemay buy into believing that there is no solution, rather than just admitting that there may be one, and she just does not know at the moment.

Being able to be in this "not knowing" space allows us to still be open to our knowing that this can heal and that we may be able to conceive, and we just don't have the answer right now. Being in this "not knowing" space allows us to have hope and possibilities. It allows us to receive direction from our source, rather than thinking we have to figure everything out by ourselves. Being in this "not knowing" space allows us to be directed from a deeper place of knowing.

There comes a time in this journey of healing that we have to be willing to be in that "not knowing" place within ourselves and continue to move forward, without any answers and without any guaranties. It's like being guided by what feels right in your heart, rather than what seems logical in your mind.

At some point during this journey, you usually reach a limit with what your minds say and then the true walking begins. It begins by moving into your heart and letting your heart guide you, by our recognition of your own deeper knowing. This deeper knowing will lead you to the healing. For this to happen, we have to be willing to tune in to our hearts and not be directly solely by our minds.

Trust Your Inner Knowing Among All Other Authoritative Voices

The Authoritative voice is the words of others that you have chosen to put all your trust in and believe, and often allow to override your own sense of knowing. It is important that all information that comes in is regarded with respect and also measured against your own knowing and sense about what is right for you. The only person that can determine what is right for you is you. You may not be the expert in western protocols, or alternative medicine for that matter, but you are the person inhabiting your body and therefore, there is an inner connection to your spirit and to your knowing of what is right for you.

Therefore, before you take for granted what someone else is telling you will work, or not work, or how things "should" be, check it out inside. Your own knowing voice is key to your healing process.

Discovering Our Truth: Statements and Beliefs That Reflect Our Truth

As we dive deeper into our mental bodies, we can explore what we think and what are our beliefs are about our womanhood. We will compare some of our beliefs against our truth statement. A truth statement is a statement that is true at the deepest part of our being; it's a statement that resonates with our hearts and our True Self.

To begin, think of two or three main thoughts, statements or judgments that come up when we think of our physical issues with our bodies. First we may feel some feelings like disappointment, or fear or hope, etc… then if we look closer there are thoughts that correspond with those feelings. Are we worried, what does the worry say? Are we terrified, what does the terror say? What does the anger say? What do these feelings say and think?

Some of us may be terrified thinking "I will never get pregnant or nothing I do will work". Perhaps, there are thoughts that say, "I will never be good enough if I am sick." All these are thoughts that contribute to your body's response to health. Sometimes these thoughts aren't too loud, so we really need to listen quietly to hear what the thoughts are underneath these feelings.

These thoughts and beliefs are not usually rational. It is an opinion someone had or you have learned and gravitated towards in your being. These thoughts may have been ingrained from generation to generation. Perhaps your mother felt she was a poor mother, she didn't meet your needs, and somehow passed those same beliefs on to you. Beliefs are passed on in the family system and unconsciously we are very loyal to them, creating conditioning in our mental field that has been passed on for generations.

But once we become aware of the operating belief behind a particular condition, we have the ability to release it from controlling us unconsciously; it becomes conscious and then we may choose. Here is one way to make your beliefs conscious.

Journaling to Uncover Our Limiting Beliefs

Now take out a sheet of paper or your journaling book. We will start our journaling process to help us break through some of these limiting beliefs.

First, take a seat and make yourself comfortable. Take a couple of deep breaths and allow yourself to focus a little on your heart. Become aware how your heart feels and breathe into this area of your body. Become aware of the difference between thinking thoughts in your head and connecting in your heart. You may do this by watching your thoughts in your mind. Become aware that there are thoughts, perhaps the thought that you are doing this exercise, perhaps you may think you do not know what you are doing, or what is the point, or maybe you have a thought that says what is next? Watch your thoughts and become aware of them, without doing anything about them, just watching.

Once you are aware of your thoughts in the moment, then place your hands on your heart and connect with your breathing… bring your focus to your heart and continue to breathe.

Now ask yourself "what do I feel about my body condition?" And see what the thoughts are that first come up for you. Write the first three thoughts down.

> For example:
> " If I have this I will never be pregnant."
> " I am not going to be a good mom, so that is why this isn't happening."
> " I don't deserve to have a family."
> " This must be happening for a reason, and there is something I have done wrong."

Sometimes it may take time to come up with the belief behind the feelings and emotions. Allow your self the time to come up with these. If you do not come up with any thoughts right away, the following may be helpful.

> What are my worries about motherhood?
> What are my worries about my body, disorder?
> What are my fears about being a woman with this problem?
> What are my fears about finance and having a family?
> How will having a child affect my marriage, career, or who I am in the world?
> What does it say about me if I have this disorder? Does it embarrass mc, make me feel shameful?

Now, focus on the first statement that you have written down. And slowly read it to yourself.

Where do you feel this in your body when you read it, in your head or in your heart?

If you feel it in your head, then put your hand in your heart, take a couple of deep breaths and ask your heart if this statement is true.

For example let's take the statement "It is useless, I should give up, I don't even have a chance to get pregnant" Say it first, recognize that it is coming from your head. Then place your hand in your heart and ask your heart "Is this true that it is useless and I don't even have a chance of getting pregnant."

Next take a deep breath and let your heart answer... let the answer come from deep inside of you... not from the previous place of concern.

The Truth statement from your heart is probably that it is not useless, and that you should be open to all possibilities. Most likely that belief of "it's useless, I should give up" is coming from a place of fear and limitation, rather than from a deeper place of wholeness in your heart.

Write the Truth statement next to the original belief. Now say the Truth statement again, which feels better in your body?

"It is useless, I should give up." Or "What I am doing does count; stay open to all possibilities."

It is obvious that the second statement sounds and feels better than the first. Feel the difference in your heart.

Breathe deeply as you repeat that message to yourself a few times, allowing it to penetrate every cell of your body.

As an extra step you may choose to write out the new statement a few times, about 10 times in your journal. This step will aid you in integrating it into your mental and physical body.

Now you may continue with another statement if you wish. Sometimes if you feel complete you can just do one statement a day, preferably in the evening or whenever you feel out of balance.

Unraveling Our Beliefs about Our Disorders

Once we have addressed some of our limiting beliefs concerning our disorders, we can also address our limiting beliefs concerning our health and any imbalances in our body.   We can begin by addressing our fear with our disorder and/or the condition of our body.

Begin by writing down our fears around our disorder or how you feel physically about your womanhood. Secondly, write what you are afraid of with this issue; for example:

I am afraid my Endometriosis will never go away and I will never become pregnant.

I am afraid that I will never have children.

I am afraid that I will never have the chance to love or be loved.

When you have written down the fears that are most dominant concerning your beliefs in your physical body, then start with the one that is feels strongest in your heart.

Breathe into your heart while you place this fear in front of you. Ask for help from a higher source than yourself, i.e.; God or Divine Light, or Divine Source, whatever you are comfortably able to work with.

As you continue to breathe deeply into your heart, watch this fear in front of you, allow it to just be there as you hand it over to Divine Essence and continue to breathe into your heart. Embrace this fear with the love and light from your heart. Light and love are from our spiritual essence, there is an endless amount. It is able to heal all emotions and physical conditions that cause pain. Call in acceptance for your condition and embrace it with love.

As you continue to breathe love and light into all this fear, there are many things that can happen. The fear changes, becomes bigger, smaller, changes from fear to anger or other emotions. Eventually it will feel different, but your job is just to hand it over and breathe the love and light that you are receiving from Divine Essence into this aspect of yourself. Watch what happens.

When you feel that the fear has changed and perhaps diminished... you can then either finish this process here or continue with the next meditation to open space for CREATION.

Allowing a New Creation
Meditation Visualization

This guided meditation is used to help us nourish our essence and prepare our body and mind to open up the space for creation.

Breathe into your heart, allow yourself to sit quietly within your heart, moving deeper and deeper into the layers of your heart. Breathe deeply into your heart, releasing tension, worries and all aspects of your day. With each breath, allow your heart to expand, connecting yourself with your source above and around you.

Allow the energy from source to enter your heart and begin to nourish your body, mind and being. Feel your body relaxing into this magnificent light, as it fills your heart with love, compassion, and healing energy.

Feel the nourishment expanding your heart. Feel yourself being carried, loved and completely taken care of. Feel yourself relaxing, opening and allowing in this source of light and essence that fills your heart and your whole being.

Now as you breathe deeply move this magnificent energy of love and light into your Solar Plexus, which is about three inches above your umbilicus.   Breathe deeply as you allow the energy to flow down and nourish your Solar Plexus.

Feel the essence filling this center, feeling your deep power, and strengthening your core deeply. Feel your beauty, your own essence filling up and expanding more and more, as you continue to breathe deeply.

Allow yourself a few minutes for this transition to take place, and fill your solar plexus completely.   Breathe and relax while your body and soul integrate the changes.

After a few minutes, allow yourself to shift your focus to your 2nd chakra. This is located right below your umbilicus, approximately 2 or 2 ½ inches below. Breathe into this area, allow yourself to see this space opening up like a flower, opening and permitting space for creation. Move the energy down from the solar plexus down to the 2nd chakra area, allowing it to fill and expand this area completely.   Feel the nourishment filling this area completely, nourishment for each and every cell to receive what it needs from source in order to be able to create and hold life. Feel this space expanding, greater and greater, as if you were breathing into a balloon.   Feel the energy flowing from the heart center of essence down to this 2nd chakra area.   Allow yourself a few minutes to continue this process.

After this has integrated into your body, start reconnecting with your heart, the true opening to all these other layers within yourself. Feel the peacefulness and tranquility within the deepest parts of your heart. Allow yourself to receive and connect your essence as you move it from your heart to solar plexus and 2nd Chakra. Feel a line of energy moving through your core center nourishing and feeding your cells and your soul, taking from the source everything you need to heal body, mind and spirit, and to move forward and to create life within yourself.

Continue to breathe and feel this line of energy immersing your whole body, expanding and providing whatever nourishment you need. Continue to allow this energy to expand until it is covering your being inside and out. Allow the expansion of it to move down your legs and into the Earth, feeling yourself releasing whatever is no longer needed. And then feel the Earth's energy coming up through your legs, supporting and reassuring your strength and power.

Allow this process to take place without having to worry about seeing it happen or understanding it, let your unconscious mind take it in and direct the changes in your body. Just relax and let it be until you feel a sense of completion for this meditation time.

When you feel complete, you may slowly start to become aware of your surroundings and bring you consciousness back to your space and time.

Remember you can do this guided meditation at anytime.

Journal Exercise: For Healing Issues of Womanhood

Take a few minutes to answer these questions in your journal. The answers will help you see your deeper meanings and beliefs around these areas.• What do you think being a woman means?• Do you feel less than a woman if part of your body is experiencing a disorder or imbalance right now? • In what ways do you enjoy being a woman?• What things make you feel less than a woman? • Write down a list of traits of being a woman that you feel you possess or should possess. Take each quality trait that you feel you do not possess, from the above list that you created, bring them into your heart, one by one and breath in their essence… ask the Divine light to help you bring these qualities into your being… sit with them for at least five minutes a day.

Journal Exercise: For Healing Issues of Motherhood

• What do you think being a female means?• What do you think being a mother is?• Do you not have a right to exist because you cannot be a mother now?• Are there other ways of mothering that you are experiencing right now in your life that you hadn't noticed until now? If yes, could you accept that you are a mother already and that you carry the mothering inside of you, regardless of your body's ability to conceive right now?

Circle the qualities of being a mother? In other words, circle the traits that you associate being a mother with, regardless of whether you feel you have these or not. You may also add your own at the end.

Cares for a group or individual

Attends to their growth

Holds others

Brings understanding

Encourages compassionate

Loving

Teaches

Guides

Creates safety for others

Strong role model

Encourages

Resourceful

Organizes the group

Shows responsibility

Dependable

Creates with her body, mind and spirit

Can You Think Of Other Qualities Of A Mother?

Now go through each one of these qualities above and bring them to your consciousness, see if you have experienced these qualities within yourself, even if you are not a mother. Let yourself see that these qualities are already within you and that you do not need to experience having the baby physically, to honor your own ability to mother. Recognize that you already carry these qualities of motherhood. See and feel each one of these qualities within your being.

CHAPTER 4

Transforming our Emotional Body

Our bodies hold emotions on a physical cellular level. Emotions are in the body and have a chemical correlation as an expression. Therefore, all emotions affect the physical body through our bio-chemistry. With all the new research in the area of neuropsychoimmunology, it has now been proven that there are chemical receptors throughout our whole body which hold certain "chemicals" that are specific to the feelings of certain emotions. Candice Pert, author of "Molecules of Emotions" 1997, states, "The chemicals that are running our body and our brain are the same chemicals that are involved in emotions. And that says to me that... we'd better pay more attention to emotions with respect to health."

What does that mean? It means that emotions are held in different parts of our bodies and correlate to particular bio-chemicals in the body. The bio-chemicals that correlate to our emotions can influence the onset of an emotion; emotions can trigger the release of particular bio-chemicals. These bio-chemicals can cause fluctuations in hormones, affect organ functions and even create muscle tension and pain. The biochemical reactions related to our emotions are a very integral factor in determining how our bodies function physiologically; they create and affect disease and

63

disorders.

If we are angry we know that our body tenses up, we may feel it in our shoulders right away. If we are overwhelmed or feel frustrated our physical body reacts to the outside stressor, thus leaving us with a physical feeling of tightness and even pain.

In the same way our mental thoughts cause a response in our physical bodies; emotional feelings can cause the same type of restriction in our system. Thus, this restriction and tension in our bodies cause lack of blood flow, nutrients and most importantly vital energy, which in turns impedes the organ system from functioning optimally and disease free.

In Traditional Chinese Medicine the emotions can weaken the organ systems and an organ system that is out of harmony can also trigger an imbalance in its corresponding emotion. One always affects the other.

For example, since anger corresponds to the organ system of the liver, a patient that is angered generally creates more stress on the liver and therefore has a higher propensity for an imbalance with the functions of the liver system, which governs headaches, migraines, body pain, painful periods, etc. We can then see the direct correlation between our emotions, organ systems and our disorders.

In turn, when we genetically inherit a kidney organ system that is deficient and not working to full potential energetically, we may have more propensities to experience psycho-emotional issues of the kidney organ system, such as fear or fearful responses, trust or lack of, and other general emotions governed by the kidney organ-system. More of the organ system and emotional correlations are explained later in this chapter.

It is important to note that if emotions affect how our bodies function, it is not so much the emotions we are feeling in the moment, but rather long standing repressed emotions that have the most impact. Emotions that have become consistent and chronic ways of expression do consistently play a large factor in our physiology. For example, if one always reacts to life events with anger or depression or a feeling of defeat, then that constant emotion will affect our physiology greatly.

On the other hand, if one is grieving an event of perhaps a miscarriage, we do not want to avoid expressing the feelings of grief, for fear of it altering our physiology negatively. On the contrary, if we do not express our grief then it goes on to be held in our cells, and our bio-chemistry unconsciously keeps responding to this inner repressed state. In this scenario it is possible to unconsciously prevent our body from becoming pregnant again. This happens as a protective mechanism in our bodies, because in essence we do not want to re-experience the trauma that has created such a state of grief. And because this grief has not been reconciled into a state of acceptance, your body's intelligence actually protects you from a perceived threat. Pregnancy can then become the perceived threat.

The good news is that it becomes a "perceived threat" and because it is perceived, it can be changed by you. So in facing the grief and allowing yourself to move through the pain and the uncomfortable feelings to a place of acceptance and resolution, then your body shifts the perceived threat to a space of allowing all possibilities available again. Therefore, you are free to conceive again, and your body completely reacts differently than how it would react previous to processing the emotion.

How We Got From Emotions To Fertility

Now, we have a new understanding of how our emotions, conscious or unconscious may be affecting our physical symptoms. Our fertility and reproductive system can be affected in this same way. If we have feelings, fears, concerns or other strong emotions from our past that have not been reconciled, it may be preventing our reproductive systems to function optimally.

Shelley's Story

There was this patient we will call Shelley. Shelley came to me with one failed In Vitro Fertilization treatment, due to poor response. She was 34 years old, and had been married for three years. Shelley and her husband both were very busy professionals. Both had busy careers and were completely immersed in their careers. Upon our first visit, Shelley expressed to me that she did not eat well, or take the time to eat; she was consumed with her work and worked until all hours of the night because it was expected for her to make her deadlines. She also further disclosed that she had been discussing with her husband the issue with their time and their lifestyles; she didn't know how she was going to fit in a baby in their schedule. She was concerned that her husband would always work until late and even if she made adjustments, she would be doing it by herself.

So even though there were some obvious nutritional issues which impeded the egg's quality and overall response of her system to create, her emotional concern had constricted her to a degree where her body was probably not going to allow a pregnancy until there was resolution with this issue of doing it alone.

In time, Shelley was receptive to suggestions on managing her time, and creating other priorities in her life, such as herself and her husband, rather than work. She also improved her food intake and the quality of the foods and conceived a healthy baby girl through natural means.

In healing it is important to explore the major feelings that surface concerning our disorders as women, in order to reconcile them and create peace and harmony within our emotional body. Peace and harmony within our emotional body creates peace and harmony within our physical body. This in turn creates health and well being. We all know that disease and disorders are states of disharmony within our being.

Sometimes, it may take time and trust to truly believe that one emotion can control so much of our outcome. But instead of doubting that belief, we can take that belief to be true and say to ourselves, "Okay, I know I am having fertility issues that are unexplained, everything seems normal, I am going to explore what other things may be affecting my body, just in case there is something that I can change." If we have exhausted our physical means, have tried western medicine, or do not want to go that route, then why not explore the other aspects of ourselves; our mental, emotional, and spiritual. What have we got to lose, we may broaden our whole new perspective about our self and our world.

Ana's Story

Ana was a patient that was very dedicated to her treatments. She came in the office with a diagnosis of "Unexplained Infertility" and both her and her husband attended treatments for more than six months. During the course of her natural treatments she also opted to do IVF treatments. Her first two IVFs failed, even though she did have embryos to be implanted, they were very low quantity. Then, a few weeks before the beginning of her third IVF cycle, Ana disclosed this memory of her childhood, when she remembered that the fear and helplessness she felt now reminded her of the same feeling she experienced in childhood, due to an aunt that wasn't able to have children. As she spent time with this aunt, she would always be consumed by this fear of ending up like her. She worried that she would fall victim to fertility issues resulting in no children, just like this aunt had? What if she was helpless just like this family member... what would she do? This stayed in her mind throughout her childhood, but was not necessarily in her everyday conscious mind.

Shortly after this process of the memory, Ana started her third cycle of IVF. Then as if by miracle, Ana's body behaved completely differently than the first two times, she responded extremely well, producing an extreme amount of follicles, which resulted in 14 embryos. Ana finally conceived and felt like her body had finally responded appropriately. And indeed it had.

Just like above, we have treated quite a number of patients that have had histories of miscarriage. The common denominators with the miscarriage cases that have received just Natural Medicine is grief. There have been variations of how people are experiencing this grief, but once they are able to be in touch with and face this place of grief within themselves; their guilt, disappointment, and fear all seem to lessen and is usually replaced with compassion, love, trust and confidence again. And even though many patients usually come to us having already processed some of their grief for their previous losses, there usually seems to be some emotional energy still lingering and some aspect of it that is still unresolved, which in turn affects their physiology and state of health.

Dialoguing With our Bodies to Reconcile our Pain

A dialogue is a conversation that we have which entails two or more voices, opinions or inputs from various sources. The dialogue we can have with our bodies will be just that, a conversation to understand better what is going on in the body and what could be done for the process of healing.

You must remember that the body has the ability to heal. When you cut yourself, the body innately has the ability to heal, and will do so without any intervention. Sometimes, if the cut is too deep, it may need some assistance from you, such as stitches or dressing for it to heal. But the actual healing process is innate; there is nothing you can do to teach the body how to heal, you can just help it do what it knows how to do.

This understanding is crucial because in dialoguing with your body, there is the understanding that the body can heal and correct itself. Furthermore, what you are doing by dialoguing is in essence removing a block that may be preventing the body from healing and functioning optimally.

Body Dialogue Connection

If you were to suspend all reservations about this process, you can dialogue with your body quite easily. But very importantly, there are a few perceptions that are necessary for you to embrace in order for this process to be successful.

- Accept that your body holds emotions in various parts.
- Accept that your heart connects you with a higher power that has all the answers within, and this ultimate power directs you to what is in your best interest always.

- Accept that your body always feels, whether you are conscious of it or not.
- Accept that your body innately knows how to heal.

Healing the Reproductive System
Meditation

This meditation is best if taped before you begin. Then play the tape
of your voice with the meditation on it. Next, find a quiet place to sit
and listen away from distractions and interruptions. This meditation
will take approximately 20 minutes.

Sit quietly and relax, as you connect with your breathing and slow
down your body and mind. Allow your breath to take you deeply
within and release any tension and stress in your body.
Acknowledge how soothing it feels to allow yourself just to breathe
for a few minutes, and relax into your breath within your
surroundings. Breathe deeply and relax. Breathe gently, relaxing
deeper and deeper. Breathe gently and relax, letting go of all the
worries, anxieties and thoughts into your breath. Let your breath
carry out all your worries and concerns. Let your breath support you
and carry you as it always has.

Now is your time, your time to nourish and nurture your body and
spirit. Let the air you breathe in soothe every cell in your body, as
you allow changes to take place and recognize that your body is able
to heal and balance. With every breath, feel the healing energy
coming into your body through your breath and fill every single cell,

providing it with the healing energy that it needs to be perfect. As you breathe in, you acknowledge that the healing energy in your breath is perfect, it is Divine, it is full of every single nourishment that is possible; it is the perfection from which all of life stems from. This energy is now being drawn into your body and each cell in your body is being immersed with this healing energy, capable of healing and balancing every need.

As you continue to breathe, allow this healing energy to move into your lower abdomen, moving through blood circulation and organs in that area. Allow this energy to fill every cell in this area of your lower abdomen. As you feel this area filling up with healing energy, allow yourself to just enjoy and relax in this energy, as it nourishes and nurtures every single part of the reproductive system that may be needed. Allow yourself to see the blood being enhanced and moving freely in this area, and the energy touching each cell and providing the necessary balancing. See each cell in this area becoming happy and receiving what it needs for perfect health from this healing energy. Allow yourself the time to breathe in and receive all the light that is needed. (Pause and breathe.)

As you continue this meditation of healing, allow yourself to acknowledge that at your core there is health and wholeness; you are nurturing your body and your reproductive system in order to create optimal health and functioning. As you relax and bring healing energy into the reproductive system, you can allow this light to cover the areas of disharmony, emotional blocks, areas of pain, fear, panic, insecurity, sadness, disappointment, grief, anger, resentment, anxiety or any other emotions, allowing them to be filled with healing light.

As you breathe healing energy into your reproductive system, allow yourself to feel and then accept without judgment these emotions being held in these areas. Then allow the deep healing light to cover them gently and accept the letting go of this pain, of the past. You may thank the emotion and images, and be willing to journal afterwards about these emotions, but for right now, you are allowing your body to release these emotions and the healing energy and light to restore your body to wholeness in all these areas. Take as much time as needed with this step. (Pause and breathe.)

As you continue your meditation of healing, continue breathing until you feel your reproductive system, uterus, ovaries and lower abdomen area completely balanced, nurtured and nourished for the day. Ask your body if there are any other areas that may be connected with the reproductive issues that need healing at this time. If the answer is yes, let your body direct you where to send the healing energy next. And as you breathe, allow the healing energy to go into these particular areas of need, relaxing them and nourishing them, restoring them to their innate state of wholeness and health. It is not necessary for you to worry about understanding the connections of these others areas of need in the reproductive system, just allow the light to continue to wash over the areas of disharmony. Continue this process until you feel complete.

And now, feeling complete and at peace, be in gratitude to your body for the wonderful messages it has given you, for allowing it to heal and shift into wholeness and be in gratitude to the light, the cosmic healing energy inherent in life itself, for allowing this wonderful healing energy through your body to create miracles and allow yourself to heal. Realize that your body has shifted into a place of peace and tranquility and wholeness, which is really your truth of who you really are. All the other emotions and mental conditions are outside of you and you need not take them in. Remember that you can always tap into this wonderful perfect space within of joy and peace and allow yourself to be nurtured and nourished when needed. Now, slowly, start acknowledging where you are, and when you are ready open your eyes, bring all the peacefulness, joy and positive attitude with you and into your daily life.

Connection to Divine Light and Source Meditation

This visualization, like all others in this book, is best if taped before you begin and then just play the tape of your voice with the visualization on it. Then find a quiet place to listen, where you will not be disturbed and you can relax for approximately 20 minutes.

Breathe deeply and relax. As you focus on your breathing, you can allow your tension and stress to melt away, soothing your mind, your body and your breath. Continue to breathe and relax, allowing yourself to breathe deeper and deeper, feeling yourself relaxing further and further. As you continue to breathe, visualize a white light entering through the top of your head, bringing it down your body, melting away all the tension and stress it encounters along the way, allowing yourself to relax even deeper. Allow the white light to travel through you and envelope you as you breathe for five to 10 cycles, deeply and slowly. (Pause.)

As you allow the breath to relax you, you can start feeling your center, your essence, your inner self. This inner self and core part of you is your connection with your wholeness and oneness, which fuels your body and mind, providing it with strength and vital force for all of its processes. Your wholeness is your true state of perfection, where everything is in perfect health and balance, where there is no lack, where there is only abundance, wellness, tranquility and peace. It's the well of life, all of life, that sustains yourself and all around you. Take a few minutes of breathing deeply as you connect with this part of yourself. (Pause.)

As you continue to breathe, you realize that your breath can connect you with this place of peace at any time. This is a practice you can do at any time. You also realize that all feelings are outside of this place of wholeness; there aren't any feelings that can penetrate this core perfect part of yourself. All feelings are outside this essence and you can gently breathe into any feelings that come up.... as you move deeper and deeper into your wholeness and oneness. As you breathe into these feelings they dissolve and allow you to move deeper into your wholeness. (Pause.)

Continue to breathe deeply as you watch the feelings melt away, and as you can feel your wholeness and sense of peace and tranquility. When you are ready, you may continue.

Next, as we move on, breathing deeply and feeling your wholeness, continue to breathe in the white light, allowing it to penetrate every aspect of your body. Realize that every cell in your body is getting nourished by this white light; allow each and every cell to receive this light. This white light nourishes every part of your body, providing exactly what the cells need.

Now take a few moments to ask your body if there is a place that needs more attention and more white light. If there is, then bring more of the white light to this area, feeling it warm and soothe that particular area, allowing it to balance and heal in whatever way it needs. If you feel complete, then you can move on to the next part.

Now before you complete this process of connection and healing, realize that your body is now centered and nourished and notice how that feels in your body. You may have feelings of tranquility, peacefulness, security, safety, where everything feels taken care of including you. Know that this feeling is the feeling of your true self, of how you can choose to be all the time. You can connect with your true self at any time, using your breath and allowing all other feelings to melt away, just by breathing and visualizing this inner core that is your truth. Now slowly, open your eyes… and you may slowly start to move around when you are ready.

This visualization may be used at anytime and should be used regularly for general wellbeing and healing.

Self Love
Meditation

NOTE: This meditation can be used for when one is feeling depleted and tired. Gathering energy of love for your body is a powerful tool to nourish physically, emotionally, mentally and spiritually. It can also be used for when one feels unloved, not good enough or undeserving and insignificant. Love really does heal everything.

To begin, lie comfortably in an area that you will not be disturbed.

Sit quietly and relax, as you connect with your breathing and slow down your body and mind. Allow your breath to take you deeply within and release any tension and stress in your body. Acknowledge how soothing it feels to allow yourself just to breathe for a few minutes, and relax into your breath within your surroundings. Breathe deeply and relax. Breathe gently, relaxing deeper and deeper. Breathe gently and relax, letting go of all the worries, anxieties and thoughts. Now is your time, your time to nourish and nurture your body and spirit. Let the air you breathe in soothe every cell in your body, as you allow changes to take place, and recognize that your body is able to heal and balance. Now, connect with your body and feel what part of your body is feeling depleted and empty. Connect with that part of your body by bringing your attention to that part. Breathe into that part of the body, visualizing your breath as energy entering that area of your body. Visualize the energy entering through your breath and filling up that area with golden white light. Continue to breathe until you feel that area full of golden white light energy. (Pause and breathe.)

As you continue to breathe, feel love in the form of golden white light surrounding this particular area of your body, from the outside, creating an envelope all around it. As you visualize this, feel the healing love energy permeate through this body area, allowing you to feel the warmth and tingling sensation in the body from the divine love. Allow yourself to feel the love, the energy and the warmth. This energy brings balance and healing to this area, raising the cell vibration to another level. Intensify the energy as you breathe and continue to love this area; this is what love feels like. Continue to feel how the love in this area feels; when it is all filled up, the sensations change, bringing a relaxed and energized feeling to the area. This healing love energy is very powerful, capable of creating necessary changes for the body to heal and receive what is necessary for its functioning.

When the area has been saturated and enough healing love energy is brought forward to it, then you may continue to spread this healing love energy all throughout your whole body, allowing your body to feel the warmth of the love and how love feels within your body. Loving yourself is very powerful and can be experienced completely by yourself, bringing the universal love energy into your body to fill any areas that may be depleted. Allow this energy to heal, nurture and nourish every cell possible. Allow yourself to heal and love all those parts of yourself that need love and wherever you may be holding unloved, unwanted residue. Allow yourself to feel the true love of the energy and how much you deserve that love. This energy of love is there for you to use whenever you need it, and it is there to fulfill you, to nurture yourself, to heal yourself and to nourish yourself. This love energy allows us to fill every inch of our bodies, allowing us to feel fulfilled, loved and taken care of. It allows our bodies to have a stronger foundation in which to function from and allow the body to heal physically as well as emotionally. This loving energy is the power within that we have that we can maximize for our wellbeing and happiness, creating great joy and peace within.

As you continue to breathe deeply, realize that you have all the means to come back and nourish yourself with this process whenever you need to. Whenever you are feeling drained, out of balance, emotional, overwhelmed or in any emotional state that is uncomfortable, this visualization will help you regain balance.

So slowly, start to realize where you are, and when you are ready, you may open your eyes, bringing with you all the positive sensations you felt throughout your session.

Aromatherapy and Self Care for Woman's Health

What Is Aromatherapy?

Aromatherapy is a term created by RM Gattefosse, a French chemist, which means "treatment using scents." It is the use of various parts of a plants and flowers in order to create an effect in the body. The body is able to absorb these fine aromatic extracts of flowers and plants and have it directly affect the limbic system of the brain. Because they work through the brain and the nervous system, these aromatherapy essences are able to initiate our innate healing responses and aid in the wellbeing of the body.

Essential oils can affect our mood, alleviate stress and anxiety, as well as help harmonize physiological processes in the body. Aromatherapy, therefore, can be used to affect changes on an emotional, mental and physical level of ourselves. The aroma can be inhaled or used in a bath, or even used on a light bulb for overall ambiance and general de-stressing effects. In our clinic, we use it directly on the body and advise patients to use it on specific points on the lower abdomen every night to assist the body in making changes.

With the help of a dear friend and a fellow aromatherapist, Mary Jean Bretton, we have created five blends that address various aspects of the feminine energy and their correlating imbalances in the physical, emotional, mental and spiritual bodies. Below are the five different formulas and what they contain.

Woman's Aromatherapy

Fire SHEN	Metal PO	Earth YI	Water ZHI	Wood HUN
Jasmine	Ylang Ylang	Sandalwood	Bulgarian Rose	Ylang Ylang
Bulgarian Rose	Juniper	Cedarwood	Sandalwood	Clary Sage
Chinese Summer Geranium	Rosemary	Patchouli	Cedarwood Atlas	Lavender
	Eucalyptus	Pink Grapefruit	Cypress	Helichrysum
	Cypress	Ginger	Jasmine	Chamomile
			Carrier Oil	Chamomile Blue

Above are the aromatherapy formulations that we created for enhancing fertility and the reproductive system. Each category has the essential oils that have been combined for that particular formula. These aromatherapy blends are used to enhance the energy in the body and help facilitate the process of fertility and wellbeing. We classified the aromatherapy formulas by the 5 Element Theory of Chinese Medicine, which is an ancient system designed by the traditional Chinese view of the world. The five-element system accounts for all the processes in our body, as well as the interrelationship of these processes in the micro and macrocosm ("Between Heaven and Earth" Harriet Bienfield and Efrem Korngold, 1991).

The five-element theory categorizes our world and the relationships within it. I have used the five elements as the classification system because it encompasses all aspects of who we are. Due to this, aromatherapy was a great match, allowing me to categorize groups of oils that would be able to address all aspects of our being and initiate the healing process within. I have chosen the five elements to be represented below by the Ancient Chinese spiritual embodiment of Hun, Po, Zhi, Yi and Shen. According to Taoist philosophy, (as written in "The Joy of Feeling- Body Mind Acupressure" by Iona Marsaa Teegaurden), "these five aspects of the psyche are essentially five ways in which we relate to life. Our feelings and emotions are messages from one or more of these five inner lands. Each is functionally related to certain parts of the body, including an organ, sense organ, body fluid and particular body parts or tissues. Each is also influenced by certain groups of acu-points. We can use these acu-points to help release physical or emotional tension and to help us contact our inner nature." Each of these elements below will detail various physical, emotional, mental and spiritual components that are related to that particular element. Use these as a guide to understand what elements need reinforcing within your own bodies and then use the aromatherapy and pressure points to balance the energy flow and strengthen that element.

Along with each element, I have created a healing message to assist in the mental healing process at the same time as you are affecting changes on the physical and emotional levels.

How Can Self Care Help?

Acupressure is the use of stimulating acupuncture points with the sensitivity of your own hands. These points that are distributed throughout the body affect change within the body, stimulating the body's innate healing ability. This healing reaction is accompanied by biochemical changes, which in turn allow stored and blocked Qi and blood to be released. The movement of the previously blocked energy (Qi) allows for more flow and energy to be circulated throughout the body, enabling the body to function optimally on the physical level.

Acupressure is an optimal way to trigger the body's healing response. This healing energy (Qi) has even been documented by western scientists through the use of microvolt meters, which are high tech electrical devices that measure energy and electrical charges throughout the body (Acupressure for Emotional Healing, Micheal Reed Gach 2004). Acupressure points are an excellent tool for releasing emotions that are held in our physical body. As mentioned before, these emotions may interfere with healing of our physical body when not addressed. By using pressure on specific points, emotions that correlate with the specific point, derived from old patterns of behaviors, are able to come to the surface and be released, allowing a freeing of Qi and blood to circulate throughout the whole body. This allows the body to have more energy for its vital processes, which in turn may be just what the reproductive area needs to enhance the fertility quotient.

That is why our emotional trauma, which we may be conscious or unconscious of, can be an important factor in our fertility issues. These emotional traumas can be stored in the reproductive area and affect our ovaries, fallopian tubes, hormones and any number of physiological functions that can and will affect our fertility. Opening up these areas using a conscious effort of acupressure and aromatherapy will help bring up these issues to be cleared and healed.

HEART SPACE DIAGRAM

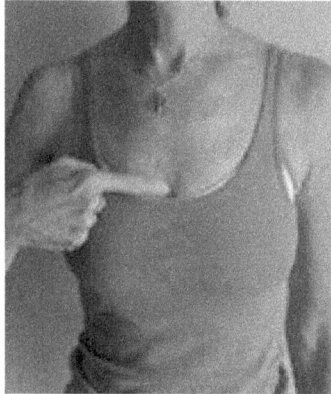

CV17

Balancing the 5 Elements with Self Care & Aromatherapy

With each element above, there are specific acupressure points to balance each of the elements and help transform emotions. Use these points with the corresponding Aromatherapy of each element by applying them on each point as indicated below.

Emotional Transformation through Spiritual Acupuncture and Aromatherapy

1. Choose a quiet location where you can sit uninterruptedly for at least 5 minutes. Close your eyes and quietly set the intention that you would like to heal your emotions today and allow light where there is pain. This intention is set by just stating it in your mind. You may also add any other particular intention you would like to receive at this time.

2. Proceed to identify the emotions that you are mainly experiencing in your life right now. You can best do this by reading each element clearly and seeing which one resonates with you the most, right now.

91

3. Continue by finding the points that correlate with that emotion and element. Find these points on your body. Proceed by applying a couple of drops of the corresponding aromatherapy on each point, pressing gently into your skin.

4. As you apply the aromatherapy to the specific points, repeat the affirmation that is part of that element, as to engage your mind in the process of letting go.

5. After completing the points on your body, proceed by using the heart light oil in the heart space (CV17 shown on previous page) to open up and allow the healing energy and light to come in.

6. Sit quietly for another minute and thank the light and source for helping you heal and connect today.

This process of clearing and transforming emotions can be done daily or even as part of a small meditation in the morning and in the evening to help start the day and clear your day. Focus on the same emotion for a few days, until you feel as if that particular emotion has cleared and lifted from your consciousness. You may have stronger emotions that may take a few days to clear or weeks, or perhaps others that may only need one day to clear.

Aromatherapy on Spiritual Acupuncture Entry Way

The following is a process to use the aromatherapy oils that are listed with each element for Fertility enhancement. Even though you still choose your Aromatherapy according to the element of imbalance, in this case you would just be applying the aromatherapy physically without needing to focus on emotions.

This may be helpful for everyday use, while the former emotional format is helpful when unproductive emotions seem to be predominant and more constant. Nevertheless, you may alternate formats as you feel necessary.

1. Lay comfortably in an area where you will be undisturbed for a few minutes. Place your hand on your lower abdomen to locate the Spiritual Acupuncture Entry Way for fertility enhancement. The entry way is located over the second chakra, or the area from below the umbilicus (belly button) all the way down to your pubic bone and covering about three inches to each side of the center. Then choose your aromatherapy according to which one you are most attracted on the previous pages.

2. Apply a quarter size of the aromatherapy on your lower abdomen and gently massage all over your lower abdomen

area.

3. Lay your hand flat on this area of your lower abdomen, providing warmth and nurturing to transmit through your hand. As you does this take deep breaths and feel yourself relaxing deeper and deeper. Bring your awareness into your heart space as you breathe deeper and deeper.

4. Then become aware of your feelings and your thoughts as you feel your hand on your lower abdomen. Try to identify the sensations in your body. Are there any feelings of sadness, guilt, anger, grief, hopelessness, helplessness, etc.? Allow yourself to feel them as you continue to use your breath to bring light to this area.

5. Continue your breathing until the light fills all and any area of pain or discomfort; physically or emotionally. Then continue to put your hand on your heart area and allow yourself to feel the peace, joy and love that comes into your heart area from Divine Source. Allow the Light to enter into your Heart space and expand into all these other areas that felt the uncomfortable feelings.

6. Embrace these uncomfortable feelings and allow yourself to breathe in loving energy from your heart into all these other

uncomfortable areas and feelings until you feel an overall sense of calm and peace in your whole body. Take your time; you have all the time in the world.

7. Breathe into the wholeness in your heart and allow that feeling of wholeness, light, love, peace and joy to expand into your whole body.....And then repeat the Healing message you had originally chosen for yourself.

For a simpler version of Aromatherapy application on areas for Fertility, you can follow the format below. This version does not release emotions consciously, but still is helpful to move blocked energy and increase healing in the pelvic area. This process will take less time and may be helpful in days when you have less energy or time to give to yourself.

Five Element Theory and The Five Cycles of Spirit

HUN – WOOD ELEMENT

Color: GREEN

The Hun is the Wood element. This is the element associated with our will, inspiration and desire for life. It is the avenue of expression that links to our source within and allows us to create from this place. Emotionally it is our ability to respond to our inner needs and create from within, rather than to attempt control of our exterior environment. An important key issue here is the acceptance of our circumstances and what the exterior world is presenting to us. Realizing that each situation may have inherent in it a gift for us, regardless of our expectation of the event, it's a huge shift of paradigm in consciousness. Only then, can we detach from outcome and control outside or ourselves and turn to creation and acceptance from within. When the Hun is out of balance, it is often expressed as depression, lack of motivation, anger, irritation and frustration. Physically we experience it as the following:

> Headaches, Migraines
>
> Pain in shoulders and neck.
>
> Pain in hyponchondriac and lower abdomen.
>
> Dizziness.

Muscle cramps.

Endometriosis, cysts and fibroids.

Painful periods or heavy periods.

Gall stones.

We can help to release emotions that are blocking the HUN phase and allow our true happiness to encompass us. The following technique, using the HUN aromatherapy oil will assist you in doing so.

EMOTIONS TO HEAL:

Depression, lack of motivation, anger, irritation and frustration.

SELF CARE:

Use the following prescription to transform the above emotions. Apply a few drops of aromatherapy on each body area, then gently rub in the aromatherapy into the indicated area for a few seconds. As you massage the aromatherapy into the particular entry areas say the following affirmation to help clear the feelings from a cellular.

BODY ENTRY AREA:

Acupressure Points: LV3, GB40.

Apply aromatherapy to the area in between the big toe and the second toe, massage well into that triangle in between the two ligaments of the toes which form a triangle. Continue to the outside of the ankle and massage all around then press the acupressure points seven times on both sides of the body.

AFFIRMATION:

I surrender to the universe's ability to respond to my needs within. I let go of Control, depression, lack of motivation, anger, irritation and frustration.

OPENING OF THE HEART:

Next use the heart oil to open up the heart and feel the love and light pouring into your being. Apply one drop of the heart oil on CV17 and hold both hands over this area as you repeat the following affirmation as many times as you feel necessary to feel a shift. Usually you will start to feel a softening, or relaxed feeling of receiving love and being supported.

HEART AFFIRMATION:

I allow my heart to open and receive the compassion and the light that we are.

HARMONIZING HUN WOOD ELEMENT

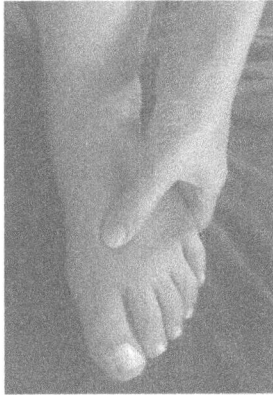
LV3

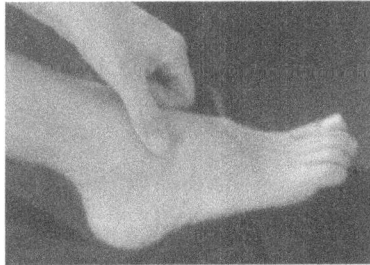
GB40

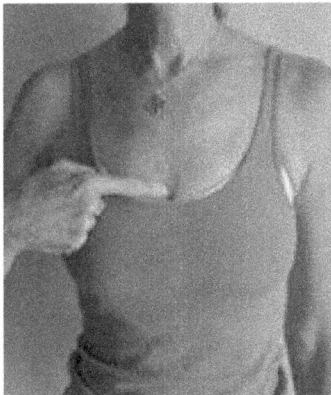
CV17

It is understandable that in reality, all the above phases interact with one another and disease on the physiological state is created by the interrelationships of these phases, not by one alone. So it is very possible that you may identify with more that one of the symptoms and emotions on various phases. Start by focusing on the most immediate feelings you experience in relation to your reproductive imbalances. For example, if you feel a sense of frustration more so than disappointment than work with the Hun phase rather than the others. You may also find it useful to alternate formulas every other day with another phase that you have identified strongly with. Asking yourself questions such as "How do I feel about my body, about being a woman, my reproductive system? And seeing which derives the strongest response...

Use your journaling from the other chapter in the areas and emotions you have identified to guide your healing process. You can also sit quietly and breathe deeply into your heart three times, then ask your Heart which phase is the best one for your healing. And listen quietly for the answer. Your heart always knows.

I would suggest not using more than two formulas at a time. If your moods and symptoms change during the course of your treatments, then change your aromatherapy accordingly.

SHEN -FIRE ELEMENT

Color: RED

SHEN is the Fire Element. It is the formula that helps to balance the energy of the Heart, passion, joy and love. The heart is one of the many entrances to our spirit and to our source of love and compassion for our selves and humanity. The imbalanced Shen is related to disconnection from our selves, our feelings of being stuck in our pain, rather than being able to move on through the pain to the truth of who we are and inability to experience our joy. When we have not been able to find joy within our hearts, we disconnect from ourselves, looking for outside people, places and things to fill us and bring us this joy. The SHEN physically affects our Hearts, Small Intestines, along with the Triple Burner and the Pericardium. Its quality is to help with overall circulatory issues and flow of fluids. Emotionally it is connected to our truth, joy and passion for our lives. When it is out of harmony, the following SHEN emotions can prevent us from connecting with our inner true state; anxiety, stress, panic, feeling nervous and on the go all the time. It is applicable for women with the following medical history:

Panic attacks

Anxiety

High levels of stress

        Insomnia

        Heart disorders

        Shortness of breath

        Nervous disorders

        Unexplained infertility

        Disorders of blood pressure

We can help to release emotions that are blocking the SHEN phase and allow our true happiness to encompass us. The following technique, using the SHEN aromatherapy oil will assist you in doing so.

EMOTIONS TO HEAL:

Anxiety, stress, nervousness, restlessness, always needing to move or do something.

SELF CARE:

Use the following prescription to transform the above emotions. Apply a few drops of aromatherapy on each body area, then gently rub in the aromatherapy into the indicated area for a few seconds. As you massage the aromatherapy into the particular entry areas say the following affirmation to help clear the feelings from a cellular level.

BODY ENTRY AREAS:

Acupressure points: HT7 and SI4.

Apply aromatherapy on inside crease of the wrist and massage, continue on the outside of the hand, the line connecting the pinky with the wrist. Then press on each point seven times on both sides of the body.

AFFIRMATION:

I am safe to connect with and feel the oneness within me.

I release anxiety, stress, nervousness, restlessness and fear and replace it with true compassion.

OPENING OF THE HEART:

Next use the heart oil to open up the heart and feel the love and light pouring into your being. Apply one drop of the heart oil on CV17 and hold both hands over this area as you repeat the following affirmation as many times as you feel necessary to feel a shift. Usually you will start to feel a softening, or relaxed feeling of receiving love and being supported.

HEART AFFIRMATION:

I allow my heart to open and receive the compassion, light and joy.

HARMONIZING SHEN FIRE ELEMENT

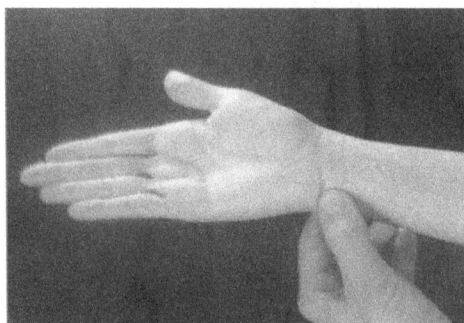

HT7

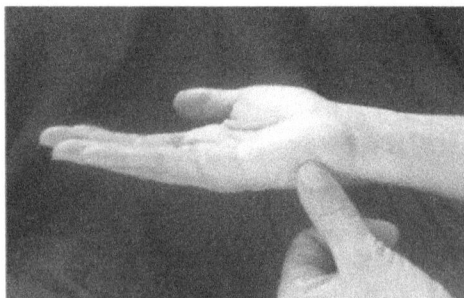

S14

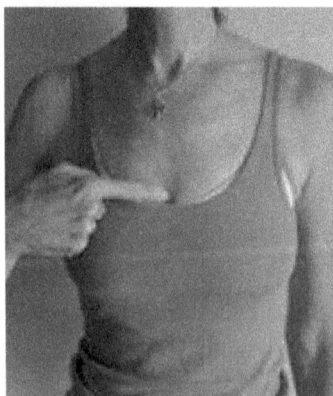

CV17

YI – EARTH ELEMENT

Color: YELLOW

YI is the Earth element. It helps us to balance the energy of giving and receiving in life. It allows us to nurture ourselves and to pass nurturing on to others. When we constantly give without receiving, or feel it is our responsibility to do everything for everyone, we do not allow ourselves to be nurtured or to receive from others. The stomach and spleen are affected when the Yi is out of balance in one self. The fluids and functioning of processing, digesting and assimilation then become slowed down and further affect our physical bodies. This is the energy that allows us to assimilate and transform nutrients, as well as emotions and events in our life. The Earth energy is associated with feelings of guilt, overdoing, too much responsibility, nervous stomach, feeling the need to nurture and take care of everyone, as well as not feeling nurtured and taken care of. It is applicable for women with the following medical history:

> Digestive issues: heartburn, bloating
> Constipation or diarrhea
> Yeast infections
> Swelling
> Cysts

Water retention

Weight metabolism

Varicose veins

PMS with lethargy, aching, and water retention

Bruises easily

We can help to release emotions that are blocking the YI phase and allow our true happiness to encompass us. The following technique, using the YI aromatherapy oil will assist you in doing so.

EMOTIONS TO HEAL:

Overdoing, exhaustion, feeling overly responsible for others and the world, over worrying, over thinking.

SELF CARE:

Use the following prescription to transform the above emotions. Apply a few drops of aromatherapy on each body area, then gently rub in the aromatherapy into the indicated area for a few seconds. As you massage the aromatherapy into the particular entry areas say the following affirmation to help clear the feelings from a cellular.

BODY ENTRY AREA:

Acupressure point: ST42 and SP3

Apply aromatherapy on top of each foot and massage, continue on the inside line of each foot, massaging the line from the big toe towards the heel. Then press on each acupressure point seven times on both side of the body.

AFFIRMATION:

I slow down and make choices that honor my body and my Self. I let go of approval, guilt, overdoing, and over-worrying, and replace it with reliance on the Divine.

I am secure knowing I am being taken care of.

OPENING OF THE HEART:

Next use the heart oil to open up the heart and feel the love and light pouring into your being. Apply one drop of the heart oil on CV17 and hold both hands over this area as you repeat the following affirmation as many times as you feel necessary to feel a shift. Usually you will start to feel a softening, or relaxed feeling of receiving love and being supported.

HEART AFFIRMATION:

I allow my heart to open and receive the compassion and light that we are.

HARMONIZING YI EARTH
ELEMENT

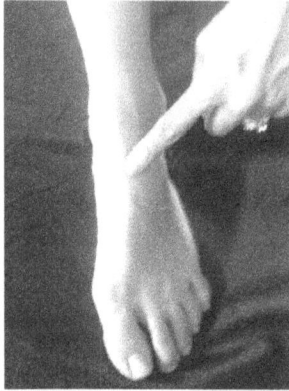

ST42

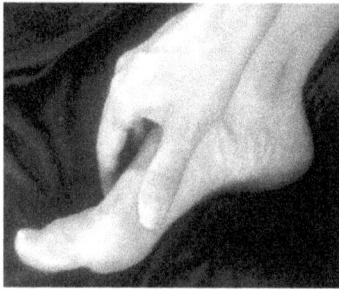

SP3

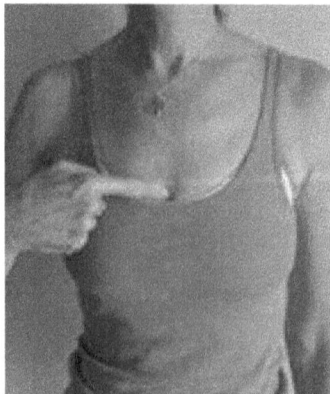

CV17

PO – METAL ELEMENT

Color: BLUE OR WHITE.

PO is the element of Metal. It represents our ability to extract from our environment what serves us, releasing what doesn't. This element is associated with the Lungs and the Large Intestines, the balance of taking in energy and resources and letting go, what doesn't serve us. The Po phase is one of transformation, in which one is able to continuously extract and release, while staying in the flow of vital energy that regenerates all of us. Feelings of grief and loneliness are connected with the lungs as well as issues of attachment and letting go. These can all be transcended by recognition of a deeper connection to the oneness of all things. By enhancing communication with ourselves we can access the truth that happiness is who we are and within rather than outside. This allows us to let go of exterior struggle with attachment, replacing it with a connection to divine flow. The Metal energy is associated with feelings of disappointment, grief, sadness, as well as attitudes of attachment, stoic behavior, and difficulty in communication. Physically, the metal element imbalances can manifest as:

Respiratory Disorders; shortness of breath, asthma, etc…

Bowel irregularities

Large intestine disorders

Dry cough

Sinus headaches/ congested nose, throat

Dry skin, nails, hair.

Lymphatic circulation issues

Breast lumps and or disorders.

We can help to release emotions that are blocking the PO phase and allow our true happiness to encompass us. The following technique, using the PO aromatherapy oil will assist you in doing so.

EMOTIONS TO HEAL:

Disappointment, grief, sadness, as well as attitudes of attachment and feeling stuck.

SELF CARE:

Use the following prescription to release the above emotions. Apply a few drops of aromatherapy on each body area, then gently rub in the aromatherapy into the indicated area for a few seconds. As you massage the aromatherapy into the particular entry areas say the following affirmation to help clear the feelings from a cellular.

BODY ENTRY AREA:

Acupressure Point: LU9 and LI4.

Apply aromatherapy on inside line connecting the thumb and the wrist, continue on the outside of the hand, on the crease area between the thumb and the second finger then press acupressure points seven times on both side of the body.

AFFIRMATION:

I allow myself to see the deeper jewel of life.

I release disappointment, grief, sadness and attachments and embrace it with love and acceptance.

OPENING OF THE HEART:

Next use the heart oil to open up the heart and feel the love and light pouring into your being. Apply one drop of the heart oil on CV17 and hold both hands over this area as you repeat the following affirmation as many times as you feel necessary to feel a shift. Usually you will start to feel a softening, or relaxed feeling of receiving love and being supported.

HEART AFFIRMATION:

I allow my heart to open and receive the compassion and light that we are.

HARMONIZING PO METAL ELEMENT

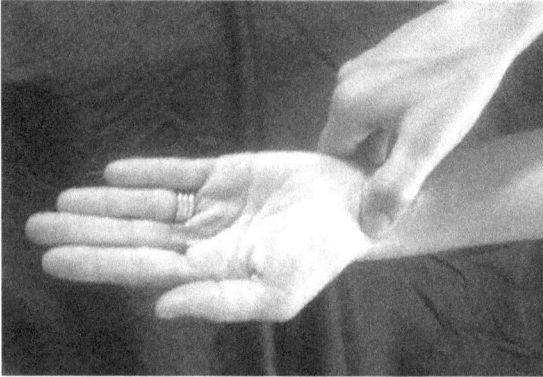

LU9

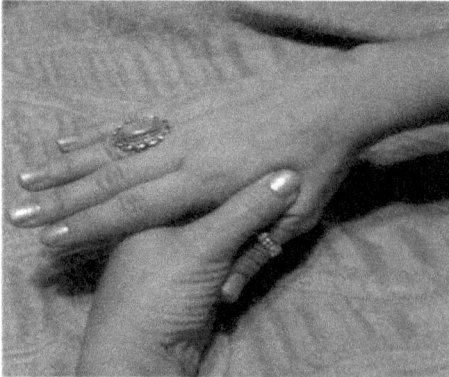

LI4

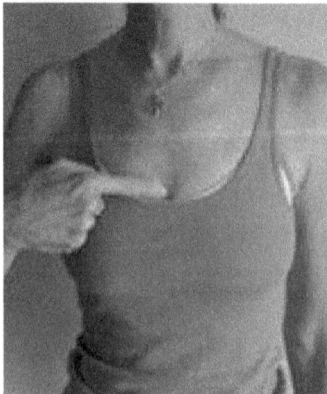

CV17

ZHI –WATER ELEMENT

Color: BLACK OR GRAY

The Zhi is the Water element. This phase is connected with our deep ability to trust in ourselves and in our deep inner power. When we lack a sense of deep trust, we experience fear and it can translate into phobias or a paranoid feeling of always expecting the worst. Knowing that we are part of a great matrix of energetic forces can lead to the trust in a greater power than ourselves which is always available to us. The Water element is driven by our insatiable quest for truth and knowledge, which liberates us from our own negative thinking and fear of life. Insecurity within is replaced by trust when we understand and have knowledge of the vast source of energy and truth that we are. These are the true qualities of our Zhi. The Water phase is associated with our kidneys and our bladder. Physiologically it can manifest as:

Urinary disorders including urinary tract infections.

Lower back pain, knee pain.

Disharmony with our spine.

Bones and bone marrow imbalances.

Tinnitus.

Infertility in general.

Egg qualities, ovarian response.

We can help to release emotions that are blocking the ZHI phase and allow our true happiness to encompass us. The following technique, using the ZHI aromatherapy oil will assist you in doing so.

EMOTIONS TO HEAL:

Fear, panic, negative thinking, terror and hopelessness.

SELF CARE:

Use the following prescription to release the above emotions. Apply a few drops of aromatherapy on each body area, then gently rub in the aromatherapy into the indicated area for a few seconds. As you massage the aromatherapy into the particular entry areas say the following affirmation to help clear the feelings from a cellular.

BODY ENTRY AREA:

Acupressure Points: KD3, BL64

Apply aromatherapy on the inside side of the foot, all around the ankle and massage, then continue on the outside of the ankle towards the outside line of the foot, all the way towards the small toe then press acupressure points seven times on both sides of the body.

AFFIRMATION:

I trust in my body's innate ability to heal.

I let go of fear, panic, terror, and negative thinking and replace it with TRUST.

OPENING OF THE HEART:

Next use the heart oil to open up the heart and feel the love and light pouring into your being. Apply one drop of the heart oil on CV17 and hold both hands over this area as you repeat the following affirmation as many times as you feel necessary to feel a shift. Usually you will start to feel a softening, or relaxed feeling of receiving love and being supported.

HEART AFFIRMATION:

I allow my heart to open and receive the compassion and the light that we are.

HARMONZING ZHI WATER
ELEMENT

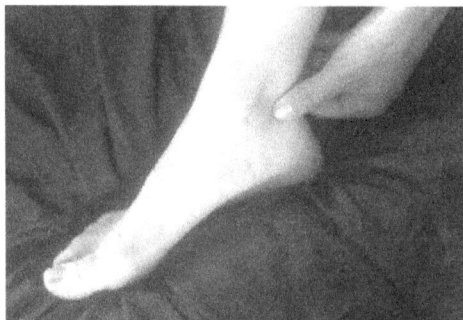

KD3

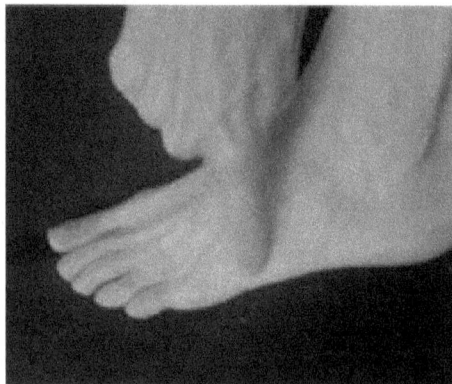

BL64

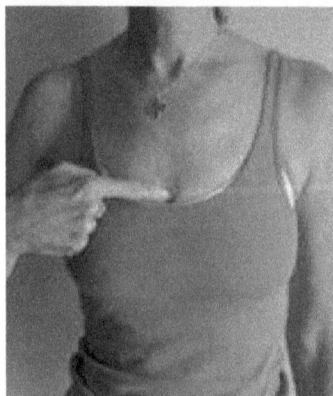

CV17

FLOWER ESSENCES

I use Flower Essences in my practice because I find them effective in helping to heal the issues relative to conception. I find Flower Essences are another modality and tool available to us that we can use to help change the vibration of our being and allow changes to occur.

Flower Essences are diluted extract of flowers and plants that are used to treat the mind, body, emotions and spirit. These essences use the same principles of homeopathic remedies in which they are diluted and potentized and made more effective than using the actual flower extract. Each liquid preparation carries the imprint of a specific plant that communicates a subtle message of healing and affects the root disharmony of disease.

On an emotional level, flower essences help harmonize negative feelings and thoughts so that you may be open to receiving change in your body. They help to transform feelings of fear with courage, feelings of resentment and anger with acceptance and motivation to act on feelings of insecurity with self confidence.

Dr. Edward Bach, the person that rediscovered Flower Essences about 60 years ago, described them in this way: "To raise our vibrations and to flood our natures with the particular virtues and to wash out from us the faults which were causing them. They are able like beautiful music or any gloriously uplifting thing which gives us inspiration, to raise our very natures and bring us nearer to ourselves and by that very act to bring us peace and relieve our suffering. They cure not by attacking disease but by flooding our bodies with beautiful vibrations of our higher nature in the presence of which disease melts as snow in the sunshine."

Even though, Dr. Bach rediscovered Flower Essences and his essences, "Bach Flower Remedies", are very powerful, I frequently use a few other companies as well. I find that times have changed in the last 60 years and some of the newer companies address emotional, mental and spiritual issues that have evolved since then. These other essences offer a different vibration and perhaps reflect our culture more accurately now. However, I still find the Bach Flower Remedies effective in many cases.

There are many ways that Flower Essences work in the physical body. The best technical explanation I have found is that of Richard Gerber MD in his book Vibrational Medicine. He states "When an Essence is ingested or absorbed through the skin, it is initially assimilated into the blood stream. Then it settles midway between the circulatory and nervous systems. There, an electromagnetic current is created by the polarity of the two systems. The Essence then moves directly to the meridians, which are vital mechanisms of interface between the subtle bodies and the physical body. From the meridians the Flower Essence is amplified out to the chakras and various subtle bodies and then back again to the physical body. The amplification also magnifies the life force potency of the Essence and aids in its assimilation. The Essence reaches the imbalanced parts of the body faster and in a more stable form. The quarts-like crystalline silica structures in the physical body, such as those in the blood stream, the hair and nails, amplify and transmit the healing energies of the Flower Essences to their appropriate sights of action, and at the correct frequencies. This whole process is similar to the way radio waves strike a crystal in a radio so that the crystal resonates with the higher frequencies, absorbing them and transforming them into audio frequencies which can be heard by the human ear.

Having said that, I have listed a few flower essences I have used with patients in my clinic. Even though I have listed them separately below, I usually test the patients using kinesiology and combine various Flower Essences together, to serve that patient in the highest way.

The Flower Essences that I most commonly use are Australian Bush Flower Essences, Fleuressences, and Bach Flower Remedies.

Australian Bush Flower Essences

ALPINE MINT BRUSH: Mental and emotional exhaustion, lack of joy and weight of responsibility of care giver. Helps create joy, revitalization, renewal.

AFFIRMATION: I CONNECT WITH MY JOY AND RELEASE THE WEIGHT AND RESPONSIBILITY OF THE WORLD FROM MYSELF.

BANKSIA ROBUR: Disheartened, lethargic, and frustrated. Helps create enjoyment, enthusiasm, interest.

AFFIRMATION: I LET GO FEELINGS OF FRUSTRATION AND DISSATISFACTION AND BRING IN ACCEPTANCE INTO MY HEART.

BLACK-EYED SUSAN: Impatience, "on the go", over committed, constant striving. Creates ability to turn inward and be still, slowing down, finding inner peace.

AFFIRMATION: I ALLOW MYSELF TO SLOW DOWN AND CAPTURE THE ESSENCE OF EVERY MOMENT.

BOTTLEBRUSH: Overwhelmed by major life changes; parenthood, pregnancy, old age, approaching death, unresolved mother issues. Creates serenity and calm, ability to cope and move on, mother-child bonding.

AFFIRMATION: AS I BREATHE, I FEEL MY STRENGTH FROM WITHIN, NOURISHING EVERY ASPECT OF MY BEING.

CROWEA: Continual worrying, a sense of being "not quite right". Creates peace and calm, balances and centers the individual, clarity of one's feelings.

AFFRIMATION: I CONNECT WITH MY PEACE AND CENTER MYSELF AS I BREATHE DEEPLY THROUGH UNCOMFORTABLE THOUGHTS.

DAGGER HAKEA: Resentment, bitterness towards close family, friends, lovers. Creates forgiveness and an open expression of feelings.

AFFIRMATION: I ALLOW MY FEELINGS OF RESENTMENT AND ANGER TO BE RELEASED FROM MY HEART, BRINGING IN FORGIVENESS AND ACCEPTANCE FOR OTHERS AND MYSELF.

FLANNEL FLOWER: Dislike of being touched, lack of sensitivity in males, uncomfortable with intimacy. Creates gentleness and sensitivity in touching, trust, openness, expression of feelings, joy in physical activity.

AFFIRMATION: I ALLOW MYSELF TO CONNECT WITH MY HEART SPACE, FEELING SAFE AND TRUSTING MYSELF.

MACROCARPA: Drained, jaded, and worn out. Creates enthusiasm, inner strength, endurance.

AFFIRMATION: I FEEL MY INNER STRENGTH AND INSPIRATION.

MONGA WARATAH: Neediness, co-dependency, inability to do things alone, disempowerment, addictive personality. Creates strength of one's will, reclaiming of one's spirit, belief that one can break the dependency of any behavior, substance or person.

AFFIRMATION: I AM CONNECTED AND SUPPORTED BY THE UNIVERSE.

SHE OAK: Female imbalance, inability to conceive. Creates the possibility of being emotionally open to conceive, female balance.

AFFIRMATION: I AM ABLE TO CONCEIVE AND CREATE.

SHE OAK W/ TURKEY BUSH: Turkey Bush – Creative block, disbelief in your own creative ability. Helps inspire creativity, creative expression, focus and ability to conceive and create.

AFFIRMATION: I AM ABLE TO CONCEIVE AND CREATE FULLY.

STURT DESET PEA: Emotional Pain, deep hurt, sadness. Creates letting go, triggers healthy grieving, releases deep held grief and sadness.

AFFIRMATION: I AM ABLE TO LET GO AND ACCEPT LOSS.

Bach Rescue Remedy

RESCUE REMEDY: Panic, distress and fear....Helps with coping.

AFFIRMATION: I AM SAFE AND CONNECTED TO MY SOURCE.

Fleuressences

Fleuressences combines various Flower Essences into a formula
which is usually more potent than using one Flower Essence by
itself. I usually combine more than one of these formulas into a
personalized formula.

(PLEASE NOTE: DESCRIPTIONS BELOW ARE WRITTEN BY
CREATORS OF FORMULA- FLEURRESSENCES)

<u>Female Balance Combination Formula</u> - there are 42 flower
essences or combinations (even more flowers!!!) in this
formula!!!! This also contains the essence of an eagle feather and
two semiprecious gems. This is a great combination for the
complicated process of being female and at the same time
evolving into a Light Goddess. This will balance hormones and
address reproductive organ issues like nothing else that I know
of. It's for anything related to being female! It helps us to be
calm, inspired, creative and lighthearted in all areas of our lives.

AFFIRMATION: I EMBRACE THE WONDER AND JOY OF
THE FEMALE ESSENCE WITHIN ME.

Self Worth Combination Formula is a blend of flower essences especially formulated to promote an improved sense of self esteem and unconditional love for our self without judgment. As the essence clears ourselves of long held negative affirmations that have blocked us from truly loving ourselves, we gain clarity about the divinity of our lives path and purpose.

AFFIRMATION: I HONOR, LOVE AND APPRECIATE MYSELF COMPLETELY.

Divine Guidance Combination Formula pulls together a wide array of essences that calm the emotions and mental chatter so that we can tune into the frequency of our intuition and higher self. This formula clears our energy field of imprints that block our ability to hear the God Self. The beauty of Divine Guidance is that decisions we make are based on information that comes from spiritual intelligence.

AFFIRMATION: I AM CONNECTED TO MY SOURCE AT ALL TIMES.

Spiritual Partnership Combination Formula is a blend of flower essences especially formulated to enhance any endeavor involving two individuals. This essence clears the energy field of long held negative affirmations that have blocked us from true spiritual partnerships on all levels. Use for committed personal relationships, business partners, or animal/human relationships. The formula can be given to animals as well. This essence reveals the divinity of each partner.

AFFIRMATION: I ACCEPT A JOYOUS RELATIONSHIP WITH MY PARTNER.

Abundance Manifestation Combination Formula is a formula that addresses the issues behind our inability to accept abundance on all levels and helps us to embrace the hugeness and ecstatic quality of being able to manifest.

AFFIRMATION: I MANIFEST ABUNDANCE IN MY LIFE.

Broken Heart Combination Formula contains 24 essences that clear negative patterns and imprints in our energy field that are related to the heart chakra. This series is for those who have had their heart broken in this life or others. This is also an important essence for those who are working on moving to greater depths in their personal relationship but have an underlying fear (often subconscious) that their heart will be broken. Sometimes we even sabotage the relationship because of this fear. This is also for those who feel that their heart is frozen.

AFFIRMATION: I RELEASE MY PAIN AND FILL IT WITH PEACE, LOVE AND JOY FOR MYSELF AND OTHERS.

Healing Ways Combination Formula is a powerful formula for assisting healers in all aspects of their work. This combination keeps us protected, centered, nurtured and healing. It is also for others for staying well and healing on all levels.

AFFIRMATION: I ACCEPT MY HEALING AND HEALTH ON A PHYSICAL, EMOTIONAL, MENTAL AND SPIRITUAL LEVEL.

How to Use Flower Essences

These Essences can be used by either choosing one formula that feels appropriate to you or choosing a few that feel like they may be appropriate. We can also create a formula that is appropriate for you in our offices, by testing you with kinesiology.

If you are choosing your own formulas, I would suggest combining SHE OAK with other formulas that feel right for you.

CHAPTER 5

Transforming from Energy to Physical Reality

Understanding Chinese Medicine and Its Application

At first sight we may only see our issue labeled as Infertility, but as we look beyond the superficial layers deeper into the pertinent levels of our existence, we can observe the interrelations that create the foundation to our being. These interrelations of our being are very important to the final equation of the physical body, even though they are less obvious and much more subtle. As discussed in the previous chapters, our emotional and mental bodies determine and influence our physical body in many ways. Now, we will continue to weave in the relationship with the physical aspect through the view of Traditional Chinese Medicine.

Traditional Chinese Medicine (TCM) is an ancient form of medicine used originally in China thousands of years ago. It is a system that stemmed from observation of the body and its symptomology and was furthered developed through experimentation with cause and effect. In other words, it was first observed then documented and theorized based on actual reality rather than on theoretical concepts that needed to be proven.

The view of Traditional Chinese Medicine incorporates the wholeness of our being. It incorporates the view that first energy is received in various ways into our body, travels through certain channels, called meridians, nourishing the organ systems and allowing optimal function. Furthermore, the understanding is that there is a range of factors that can affect this energetic flow, which may impede our organ systems from functioning optimally. Things like emotions, our nutrition, our genetics, our daily practices, our mental practices, our stress, and many more can all interrupt this flow of energy and start the downward spiral of deterioration and disease. In TCM the body is made up of the interaction of the whole and basically what we have been talking about in this book.

For our purposes we will narrow this vast subject of Traditional Chinese Medicine into a couple of categories only. The first will be the five elements which have been discussed earlier in Chapter 3 and the general physiological imbalances relating to fertility with the accompanying Herbal formulas.

Traditional Chinese Medicine, as discussed in Chapter 3, describes this interrelation of our energetic flow, through the explanation of the five elements. These five elements include not only the emotional correlations, but also group organs, colors, smells, actions and even particular archetype for each element. For a detailed description, read "Between Heaven and Earth"- A Guide to Chinese Medicine, Harriet Beinfeld and Efrem Korngold.

Now we can take a look at the patterns of disharmony that may cause the imbalance in the reproductive system or what may show up as "Infertility". Regardless of whether the western diagnosis is Endometriosis, Luteal phase defect, Hormonal issues, Egg Quality, Polycystic Ovaries, Tubal Blockage, or even Unexplained Infertility, the underlining patterns in TCM are diagnosed slightly differently.

Infertility in TCM is a symptom which tells us that there is disharmony in the reproductive system which may be either obstructed or affected by other functions in the body. According to TCM, there are numerous dysfunctional patterns that can cause infertility. We will start with two major groups; Deficiency and Excess.

Deficiency basically means that the cause is depletion in some aspect or not enough of something. It may be self produced due to overdoing, not enough nutrients or not enough of the ones needed, or there may be a genetic deficiency to begin with. The deficiency can be of Qi (vital energy), Yin (fluids), Yang (vital heat) Blood or Essence. Each organ system has to maintain a delicate balance within these four factors in order to maintain the integrity of the system and its health, and to avoid deterioration and disease.

An Excess condition is when one of these aspects; Qi, Yin, Yang, or Blood; have accumulated and have created blockage. This blockage may result in accumulation such as fibroids, endometriosis, or fluid retention, to name a few. Excess conditions prevent the harmony of an organ system or various organ systems to function properly by blocking the continual flow of these substances named above and slowing down the system.

Now, Deficiency is easy to understand because we all have felt exhausted in our daily life or at some moment if not at all. In our society we feel the pressure to perform and do more, and this condition of exerting more than we have time to fill within ourselves definitely causes us to exhaust and deplete ourselves.

On the other hand Excess is a little differently. Excess happens for example, when our systems do not process our fluids well (spleen and stomach imbalance), and there is an excess of fluid accumulation which turns into excess fluids (dampness) aggravated perhaps by a wet and cold environment, then can affect our "lower burner" which will affect Fertility.

In truth there are few conditions that I have seen that are purely excess or deficiency alone. Most conditions have a combination because it is natural for the body to have deficiency and excess at the same time. I will explain. For example, if you have Blood deficiency in which you feel tired, dizzy and have dry hair and nails, then the blood in the organism is low of quantity and perhaps quality, in some areas of your body your circulation will be affected and therefore because there isn't enough, as your circulation slows down, certain areas may have less momentum and pool together, starting to cause what we would call a stagnation, and more accurately a stasis because it is blood, rather than Qi. So now you have an area of excess (blood stasis) and a deficiency (blood deficiency) at the same time.

This scenario is very common in fertility cases. In the above case you would have to take into consideration the deficiency in order to balance the organism, because if you would just resolve the stasis, and not build up the blood (nourish blood), then the quality of the patient's condition would not improve much.

Many things influence these deficient and excess conditions. Our systems respond to our emotional and mental stimulus for one. Then we also have the affects of our ancestors and hereditary factors to consider. What we received at birth sets the stage for what our weak links are going to be. Our environmental factors are our next group of factors to consider.

Where we work, how we work, what we spend our day thinking about and feeling, these continuously are the input for the cells to be built from. Other factors include how we react to our environment and our personal scripts and beliefs. Are we constantly worried and scared, this will affect our Spleen and Kidneys. Are we trying to control everything outside of ourselves, or constantly feeling angry and frustrated? This will affect our liver and gall bladder. These correlations were written in the five elements segment in Chapter 3.

Other environmental factors to consider: the weather, the coldness or heat or dampness or wind factor, these all contribute according to Traditional Chinese Medicine. Nonetheless, even though we cannot control our weather, it is important to realize that all the other factors we can shape and mold with a little bit of focus, energy and patience. We can start to take real control from within as to our responses to our environment, as well as create our bodies from our conscious choices rather than our subconscious reactions.

In other words, when we start to take the time to reframe our mental thoughts, take notice and apply some meditations to shift how we feel all the time, we then start to make conscious choices in our everyday interactions rather than just continuing to react from our old script and from the messages that we learned when we were young. We stop reacting from our storage in our brain, and make choices that serve us now, where we are right now in our lives. Sure, it takes time to reevaluate what we are doing, how we are reacting, what is bothering us, and what we are feeling. But it also allows us to choose and have control over our self and our life, rather than feeling helpless and unhappy.

Now that we know what influences our body, let's look at some of the patterns in TCM that are common to Fertility. First a brief review of Excess and Deficiency patterns.

Excess

Excess syndromes are seen as disorders such as endometriosis, fibroids, cysts, or any accumulation, mass or tumor. Most of these conditions also have a deficiency factor to them. In Excess patterns, there is always something that is building up or stagnating. This accumulation is of Qi, blood, phlegm or damp. Sometimes the accumulation happens because the system as a whole is very weak and the Blood may not move, and it starts to back up and create mass in certain areas. Sometimes the fluids are not processed properly by the Spleen and Stomach system and then they start to accumulate causing Phlegm/Damp Accumulation. So in many cases

Excess conditions are furthered complicated by a deficiency factor as well.

Deficiency

Deficiency conditions are seen in many disorders such as hormonal imbalances, unexplained infertility, miscarriage, low responder, low sperm count and others. Endometriosis, fibroids, cysts, or painful periods, etc., may also have a deficiency imbalance as a secondary factor. Deficiency conditions are due to the organ systems operating too low in Qi, blood, yin, yang or Essence. When an organ system is deficient it does not have the strength to function properly and in turn affects the next organ that is dependant on it. This causes a reaction in the body of imbalance and it further aggravates symptoms.

According to Giovanni Maciocia in "Obstetrics and Gynecology in Chinese Medicine, he says "In cases of Deficiency, the Uterus and the Directing and Penetrating Vessels lack the necessary nourishment to nurture and fertilize the egg; in the case of Excess, pathogenic factors obstruct these structures and prevent their proper Qi, Blood and Essence transformation so that the fertilization cannot occur." Furthermore, one study that was reported by in Beijing's Journal of Chinese Medicine, of 257 cases of Infertility, (as summarized by Maciocia) showed the percentage of the patients that fell into the following patterns of differentiation of Chinese Medicine.

Kidney Yang Deficiency: 27.63%

Spleen and Kidney-Yang Deficiency: 12.84%

Liver and Kidney Yin Deficiency: 11.67%

Kidney Yin Deficiency with Empty Heat: 5.06%

Liver Qi Stagnation: 7.39%

Blood Stasis: 29.57%

Phlegm: 3.11%

Cold Dampness: 2.73%

The patterns of differentiation of Traditional Chinese Medicine will be described later in this chapter.

What are these Organ Systems? Organ systems are each of our organs, such as the Liver, Kidneys, Heart, Stomach; Spleen etc... with all of the corresponding meridians and channels, as well as all of their related functions. Each organ system is responsible for certain functions in the body due to its meridian and channel relationship and physiology in the body. The Kidney organ system, for example is responsible for lower back and knee function, urinary disorders, slow bone growth and development, sperm motility- low count and mobility issues, low libido, and general fertility, to name a few. In TCM the organ system is categorized as not only the organ itself, but also with the functional aspects that it is responsible for.

Many disorders involve more than one organ system in the body. When one organ system is out of balance, the rest of the body will have to compensate for that disharmony and through the process of compensation other organ systems lose their stability as well. Most Infertility issues are related to the Kidney organ system, but also may have a Liver organ system disharmony resulting in excess headaches or migraines, extreme mood swings along with irritability, and there may also be a Heart organ system disharmony resulting in Insomnia, restlessness, high levels of anxiety,and even including palpitations and panic attacks.

As you see, the body is a myriad of functions, each one affecting the other. Below is a list of the organ systems and their related functions, so that greater understanding of your body will hopefully lead to the enhancement of fertility.

Relationship of Symptoms and Patterns

A person who is experiencing infertility, headaches, night sweats, pain with the menses, and lower back pain may feel that all these symptoms are unrelated in the body. In fact, they are extremely related and the ROOT CAUSE of the problem may be the same. It can be due to a liver or kidney deficiency for example, an acupuncture physician works with this person to treat the deficiency, the person will see all the symptoms improve. This is the beauty of TCM, that all these seemingly unrelated issues have a connection. And so with this we can understand our body and how it works.

Below I have outlined some familiar patterns that I have seen in my Fertility practice, along with some of the western diagnosis that are familiar within these patterns. Please note that a person may not experience all the symptoms in order to have that particular syndrome or deficiency. Sometimes you only experience one or two of the symptoms. Also note that when it comes to the western diseases such as Endometriosis for example, there may be more than one syndrome or pattern that can cause these imbalances.

Below you will find some of the most common observations for the causes of Infertility that I have seen in my patients. This chart can give you an idea of what are the most common causes that are seen with each disorder. Although these are just a sample of what most patients have shown in clinic, it does not mean that it can be the only diagnosis or necessarily the correct one for you.

PHYSICAL DISORDER	CORRESPONDING IMBALANCE
Ovulation; Absence or irregularity:	**Kidney Yang Deficiency.** **Kidney Yin Deficiency.** **Blood Deficiency.**
Blockage of Fallopian Tubes:	**Damp Heat or Dampness in the Lower Burner.** **Blood Stasis.**
Pelvic Adhesions:	**Dampness with sometimes LV Blood stasis.** **Kidney Deficiency.**
Endometriosis:.	**Blood Stasis.** **Blood Deficiency.** **Kidney Deficiency.**
Uterine Myomas, Fibroids, cysts:	**Blood stasis.** **Blood Deficiency.**
Low Responder & Poor Quality of eggs	**Kidney Jing, Kidney Deficiency.** **Blood Deficiency.**
Polycystic Ovaries:	**Dampness in Lower Burner** **Kidney Deficiency.**
Unexplained Infertility:	**Kidney Jing.** **Kidney Deficiency, Yin & Yang.**
Hormonal Imbalances:	**Kidney Yin.**
Low Progesterone	**Kidney Yang.**
Miscarriages. History of:	**Kidney Jing.** **Kidney Yang.**
Infrequent or No menses.	**Blood Deficiency.**

Additionally, most patients that experience a combination of disorders may also have a combination of core imbalances taking place. There may be, for example, Dampness in Lower Burner with Blood Stasis when a person is showing Blockage of Fallopian Tubes and Endometriosis. For that reason, please use the chart below to show the commonalities of the disorders, but not specifically for diagnosis of your own situation.

Understanding Chinese Medicine Substances

Following is a brief synopsis of each of the key substances used in Chinese Medicine. This substance describes the processes of the reproductive system and also adds insight into its dysfunction.

Kidney Jing

The first substance is Jing. Jing is translated as reproductive essence. It is inherited from our parents and stored in the Kidneys, therefore referred to as Kidney Jing. The quality of Jing determines our genetic tendencies and predispositions. The quality of our Jing establishes to some degree our basic constitution, also known as our hereditary factors. If our Kidney Jing is strong then there is more likelihood that we will be able to have children and pass it on. Jing deficiency manifests as:

- Primary amenorrhea
- Poor ovarian quality
- Intermittent and sporadic cycles (oligomenorrhea).
- Delayed puberty
- Premature menopause
- Poor or no response to fertility drug treatments.
- Sterility
- Weak constitution
- Unexplained Infertility
- Small uterus or ovaries

Our Kidney Jing also known as essence, declines with age and with many other factors, thus that is why our fertility declines naturally with age. For example, it gets used up by the hundreds of menstrual cycles that women experience, as well as life style and demands we put on ourselves. The decline of Kidney Jing is also the reason more miscarriages occur and that more genetic disorders are common in women that are older.

Kidney Jing is however able to be treated and even though it cannot be reversed completely; it can be enhanced through Herbs and acupuncture. It can be improved enough to have a significant positive outcome on a patient with a history of miscarriages, or even with a patient that has responded poorly to western Fertility treatments in the past. With a little persistence and consistency over a significant length of time, Kidney Jing can be improved.

Kidney Yin

Yin is the term to describe the cooling, nourishing and moistening substance and internal aspect of body function and structure. In reproduction, Kidney Yin relates to the hormonal triggers which stimulate follicles to develop and support the follicles growth and maturation. Kidney Yin would also involve the pituitary's function within the process of hormonal triggers.

Kidney Yin controls the lining of the uterus and its secretions thus having the growth of the lining dependant upon the quality of Yin. This is critical in addressing patients with a decreased lining which prevents successful implantation of the Uterus. Some of the common symptoms that may be seen with Kidney Yin Deficiency are:

- Scanty production of vaginal and cervical mucus.
- Scanty ejaculation.
- Thinner uterine lining not capable of maintaining pregnancy.
- Scanty periods.

- Poor growth of follicles.
- Ovulation delayed or too early.

As above with Kidney Jing, the Kidney Yin can be enhanced to an even greater positive degree. Kidney Yin usually responds faster than Kidney Jing when treated with regularity and consistency. Yet, Kidney Yin can also be damaged by excessive activity with little rest, overwork, excess sexual activity, as well as a weak constitutional tendency from birth.

Therefore it is important that changes in our lifestyle are incorporated into the complete protocol of nourishing Kidney Yin and that proper rest of the physical body as well as the mind be integrated for real changes to occur. When nourishing Kidney Yin, meditation practices are essential to the healing process.

Kidney Yang

Yang is the dynamic, active and warming effect in the body, and it is mostly felt during the ovulation process. The journey of the egg down the tube is also a dynamic one, with both egg and tube requiring smoothness and flexibility which Yang provides. Yang ensures mucus obstructions in the tube are dissolved and the tubes are free flowing, to allow passage of the eggs. Yang also is the motivational force for all transformations in the body, such as ovulation and conception.

The process of fertilization also relies on sufficient Yang, as the sperms head finally breaks through the egg's coating and its DNA fuses with that of the egg, which is the greatest transformation of the all.

Cold Uterus is a description of deficiency of Yang in the Uterus, which prevents an embryo from implanting in the uterus, and it is also considered to have insufficient progesterone which creates coldness in the body.

Kidney Yang deficiency may be caused by:
- constitutional tendency
- result from damage invasion of external cold in through the particular channels;
  - Stomach channel -eating cold foods like ice cream.
  - Uterus channel- by swimming in chilled water during the time of menses.
  - Channels on the legs – by wearing scanty covering on your legs, during the time of menses.
- Emotional constraint may also cause Kidney Yang deficiency because Kidney yang is designed to move and be

free and when we repress and suppress emotions it affects our Liver and Heart Qi, which in turn damages the Kidney Yang.

- Lack of sleep will also damage Kidney Yang.
- Miscarriages, abortions, and thyroid disease.

Kidney Yang is treated in the post ovulation phase of the menstrual cycle with herbs and acupuncture which helps to boost Kidney Yang. This treatment will also help to increase progesterone production, increasing fertility overall.

It is important to note that in order for Kidney Yang to improve sleep patterns must be harmonized and improved first.

Blood

As we noted in the original diagram, Blood is associated with a lot of the syndromes and imbalances in fertility.

The Blood in Chinese medicine include more than just the blood in the arteries and veins; it includes aspects of tissue nutrition. The Heart governs Blood and the Spleen plays a role in the production of blood; therefore both these organs contribute to the production and quality of the Blood. In fertility, Blood nourishes the endometrium making it nutritious for the embryo to settle in. Shortly before ovulation, peaks of estrogen released by the developing egg, primes the lining of the uterus, this means the endometrial tissue is provoked by this hormone in to proliferation and growing in size, actually producing more blood vessels and laying down more tissue. Therefore, Blood (not just Yin) can delay ovulation.

Blood is stored by the Liver, when the body is at rest. This must be passed on to the Uterus before preparation for pregnancy or menstruation can occur. So if the Liver Blood is deficient, then menstruation may be scanty or there may be infrequent or no periods.

Blood Deficiency can cause:
- Scanty or infrequent periods.
- Late ovulation or no ovulation
- Miscarriages
- Low responder to Fertility Drug Treatment – Poor quality of eggs.
- Endometriosis.

Blood Deficiency is caused by:
- Inadequate consumption of protein.
- Heavy periods also exhaust the blood.

- Constitutional tendency to anemia.

Blood Deficiency is treated by using adequate amount of protein and iron in the diet. Building up the Blood is emphasized in the weeks immediately after the period.

Shen

Shen translates to spirit and encompasses the deeper spiritual levels and virtues, as well as the brain and nervous system. Shen is related to and controlled by the Heart. The Shen and the Heart play an integral role with the Kidneys in controlling fertility.

Healthy Shen and Heart will create mental stability and contentment. Ovulation relies on the Heart housing the mind or (Shen). When the Heart and Shen are stable, the cues for the different stages of the menstrual cycle can proceed smoothly. Emotional stress can disrupt the menstrual cycle, affecting the disruption of the hypothalamus, causing the pituitary gland dysfunction, and ovulation may be delayed or completely switched off.

Shen also balances the Kidney Yin and Kidney Yang and maintains the healthy harmony between both of them, insuring the transformation of one to the other, which is a critical process for ovulation and conception to take place. In other words, if Kidney Yin does not transform into Kidney Yang due to obstructed Heart Qi(caused by emotional stress), then ovulation will not occur.

Shen instability is treated by first treating the stress of the person as well as the mind. Regulating sleep patterns is crucial as well as removing mental stressors and employing tools for reflection, meditation and relaxation. Treatment for Shen instability can be applied at any time, and can be emphasized especially in the days leading up to ovulation.

Chinese Herbology to Enhance Fertility

Chinese Herbology is the use of whole plant/animal substances to treat the root organ system of the body, as well as the symptom the patient is experiencing. Chinese Herbology differs from western drugs in the sense that the approach in Herbology is that of using a whole substance instead of the western pharmacological approach of taking a plant substance and extracting the most effective molecule for a certain disease.

Using a whole substance has been proven to be safer and treats a variety of ailment in a gradual natural way, healing the body along the way. An extracted molecule is more aggressive, with side effects that can be dangerous and does not necessarily create healing by creating health, but rather just diminishing the clinical symptoms of a disease.

Nonetheless, no one argues that western drugs are highly efficient in certain cases of urgency, yet by far, natural herbal approach is an overall healthier and safer approach to treating and healing the body. It is an approach in which the whole product is able to be absorbed slowly into the metabolism and has success on a broader, more gradual scale, because the plant itself has other ingredients which offset the side effects. The Chinese pharmacopeias is one of the most extensive in the world and have been used for more than 3000 years in internal medicine and especially with women's health. Following I have added some formulas for treating each organ pattern.

Pattern Differentiation Affecting Fertility

In addition to the substance description in the previous page, I have written brief descriptions of the patterns of differentiation according to imbalances in the body overall, with an emphasis on the reproductive cycle along with a Chinese Medicinal Herb formula that would be applicable. Please note there are many formulas that may apply, I have only given these as examples, but they are by no means the only formulas that are available.

Deficiency Patterns

Kidney Yang Deficiency

Prolonged menstrual cycle, the period could be either scanty or heavy and dull in color, along with cramps that feel better with heating pad or heat, lower back pain, dizziness, feeling cold, depression, frequent urination, low libido, often fearful, early morning loose urgent stools.

Herbal Treatment for Kidney Yang Deficiency

Ba Zhen Yi Mu Tang : This formula is particularly indicated if in addition to a deficiency of Kidney-Yang, there is a pronounced deficiency of Blood. Herbs are added to move Qi and invigorate Blood to counterbalance all the tonic herbs in the formula.

You Gui Wan: This formula is for Kidney-Yang deficiency and essence deficiency as it supplements the Kidneys and warms the Yang.

Kidney Yin Deficiency

Infertility for a long time, lower back pain, soreness or knee pain; ringing in ears or tinnitus; ovulation cervical mucus is scanty or missing; periods are early, scanty with light colored blood; night sweats, dizziness, hot flashes, thirsty.

Herbal Treatment for Kidney Yin Deficiency

Yang Jing Zhong Yu Tang- This formula tonifies the Kidneys, nourishes the Essence and Blood and promotes fertility.

He Che Da Zao Wan – This remedy nourishes Kidney-Yin and Blood.

Zhi Bai Di Huang Wan: This formula tonifies Kidney-Yin and cools deficiency heat.

Blood Deficiency

Menses are scanty or late; pale blood, tiredness, depression, dizziness, dry flaky skin, fingernail and toenail brittle, diminished night time vision; blurred vision, pale complexion.

Herbal Treatment for Blood Deficiency

Ba Zhen Tang – This formula tonifies Qi and nourishes Blood.

Heart Deficiency

Wake up early in the morning and have trouble getting back to sleep, heart palpitations, nightmares, tend to feel agitated or extreme restlessness, prone to panic attacks.

<u>Suan Zao Ren Tang</u> – Nourishes the Heart, calms the Spirit and nourishes Liver Blood.

<u>Tian Wan Bu Xin Tang</u> – Harmonizes the relationship between Heart and Kidneys.

Excess Patterns

Cold In Uterus

Primary Infertility, delayed cycle, scanty period, small clots, painful period, better with heat, feeling colder during period, pale face, feeling cold, sore back. This is more common in young women.

Herbal Treatment for Cold In Uterus

<u>Ai Fu Nuan Gong Wan</u> – This formula nourishes Blood, tonifies Kidney-Yang, and expels Cold form the Uterus.

<u>Wen Jing Tang</u> – This formula expels Cold, nourishes Blood, clears Empty (Deficient Heat) from Blood Deficiency.

Stagnation of Liver Qi

Irregular periods, pre-menstrual tension (pms), painful periods, breast distention, elevated prolactin levels, bloated during or before menses, menstrual blood thick and dark or purplish in color; prone to irritability, depression, anger or frustration.

Herbal Treatment for Stagnation of Liver Qi

<u>Xiao Yao San</u> – This formula moves Qi and tonifies Spleen Qi, pacifies the Liver and nourishes Blood.

Blood Stasis

Irregular or painful periods, dark blood with clots, mid cycle pain around ovaries, painful breast lumps, periodic numbness of hands and feet, varicose veins, cherry red spots on your skin, lower abdomen tender to palpation, mental restlessness, tend to be irritable.

Herbal Treatment for Blood Stasis

<u>Shao Fu Zhu Yu Tang</u>- This formula invigorates Blood, eliminates stasis and expels Cold.

<u>Wu Jin Wan</u> – This formula invigorates Blood and eliminates stasis.

Dampness in the Lower Burner

Irregular periods, delayed cycle, mid-cycle pain, vaginal discharge, long term infertility, adhesions, prone to obesity, feeling of heaviness, feeling sluggish after meals, prone to yeast infections or vaginal itching, joint aches and pains, fibrocystic breasts.

Herbal Treatment for Dampness in the Lower Burner

<u>Qi Gong Wan</u>- Resolves dampness in lower burner.

DAMP HEAT

Early periods up to twice a month; Heavy flow, feeling hot during period, foul smelling vaginal discharge, vaginal or rectal itching during your premenstrual phase, thirst, mental restlessness.

Herbal Treatment for Damp Heat

<u>Si Miao San</u> –Resolves damp heat in the lower burner and the genital system.

Organ/System Clinical Symptomology

Below are symptoms that are classified by their respective Organs which are responsible for the proper function of these aspects of your physical body. I include these categories here, so that you are able to understand the correlation between your symptoms and the deeper root organ system, therefore making better sense about these seemingly separate symptoms.

Each organ system is responsible for certain functions in the body, not just physiological ones but also psycho-emotional responses.

Below are the main organ imbalances and their corresponding symptoms. Only the most common imbalances have been included. This list below is not a complete representation of Traditional Chinese Medicine organ systems.

Heart Organ and Channel Imbalances

Feeling anxious and stressed out, feeling nervous, palpitations, panic attacks, chest pain, insomnia, dream-disturbed sleep, restlessness, poor memory, circulatory and other cardiovascular imbalances, pain in the eyes, pain on the inner side of the arm and pain along the scapula.

Lung Organ and Channel Imbalances

Feeling melancholy, sadness, excess feeling of grief, not being able to take in life, coughing, excessive colds, asthma, chest distention or pain, tired feeling in the daytime or morning, and other respiratory imbalances. Fever, aversion to cold, stuffiness of the chest, pain in the clavicle, shoulders and arms.

Spleen Organ and Channel Imbalances

Excess worrying, feeling excessively out of control or in need to be in control, excessive thinking, lethargy after eating, poor appetite, crave sweets, easily bruised, nausea, abdominal distention and bloating, diarrhea or loose stool, heartburn, sluggishness, edema and other gastrointestinal imbalances. Vaginal discharge, cold feeling along the channel, weakness of the leg muscles.

Liver Organ and Channel Imbalances

Feeling on edge, irritable, overwhelmed, excessive planning and control, angry and frustrated, depression, resentful, hypochondriac pain, headaches, migraines, muscle spasms, menstrual irregularities, dysmennorhea, endometriosis and other hepatic disorders. Headache, pain and swelling of the eye, cramps in the legs.

Kidney Organ and Channel Imbalances

Fear and doubt, hopelessness, lack of will, lower back and knee pain, dizziness, ringing in ears, urinary disorders, low sexual libido, premature gray hair and kidney imbalances. Pain in the soles of the foot.

Stomach Channel Imbalances

Pain in the eyes, epistaxis, swelling of neck, facial paralysis, cold legs and feet.

Large Intestine Channel Imbalances

Sore throat, tooth-ache, epistaxis, runny nose, swollen and painful gums, swollen eyes.

Small Intestine Channel Imbalances

Pain in the neck, pain in the elbow, stiff neck, pain along the lateral side of the arm and scapula.

Bladder Channel Imbalances

Fever and aversion to cold, headache, stiff neck, pain in the lower back, a pain in the eyes, pain behind the leg along the channel.

It is important to note that while the Kidneys and Liver system are more closely related to gynecological disorders in Traditional Chinese Medicine, other organ systems also contribute greatly and are usually involved even though they may not be directly the core cause.

Feminine Wisdom: Rise to A New Creation

CHAPTER 6

Transforming the Physical Body

Nutrition/Biochemistry

Nutrition is the foundation of our body's health system. What you put in your body is as vital as any other factor in enhancing fertility. So while our emotions and our mind have a great deal of dictation in creating the state of our health, what we eat is also a key element in the outcome of our physical condition. Food choices are building blocks and affect our energy, our state of health and what we create from this state of health.

Imagine that you make great changes in lowering your daily stress; you make progress in your physical symptomology through meditation, etc., but then continue to eat foods that do not honor your body's highest level of health and functioning. Your positive conditions of health cannot last, because you are not building a solid foundation from which the body can sustain itself.

Your physical body is largely made up of what you put into it. If you eat foods that are laden with chemicals and have very little nutrients, your body cannot receive the necessary nutrients to build healthy outcomes. Where will these nutrients come from? Taking a vitamin does not cover all the bases of nutrients. There are many nutrients inherent in food that cannot be replaced by a supplement. When foods are taken out of their natural context of which nature has grown them in and we isolate a compound from a particular food source, the body cannot duplicate the natural environment that product was alive in, which in turn affects the ability for the body to absorb that particular nutrient.

Nature creates in a particular order, for example; vitamin a is derived from beta-carotene, which is derived from carrots. Your body benefits more from carrots and betacarotene than from the isolation of Vitamin A. This is because in its natural environment, the actual food source has many other compounds that help us absorb and digest the nutrients within. When we isolate a compound it may be missing the essential nutrient found in nature that gives that particular compound the maximum benefit.

Therefore, it is always more beneficial to drink vitamins and nutrients that are found in their natural environment as much as possible. In other words, it is better to digest vitamins made from a whole food, rather than isolated ingredients in a laboratory.

Eating foods that lack in nourishment will contribute to Deficiency conditions in our bodies, while eating foods that are too acidic on the pH scale will cause Excess conditions in our body. Some foods cause stagnation and others contribute to blood stasis or heat conditions in our bodies. Many foods contribute to an inner environment of toxins and a perfect terrain for symptoms of disease to occur. Our pH balance and the balancing of our foods are keys to maintaining our inner bio-chemical balance and our healthy foundation.

The biochemistry of our organ systems is an integral part of a wholistic program, because without it, health and healing in the body can not be sustained and realized for any real length of time.

In a deficiency case, a person that is depleting themselves by the quality of food they are eating is basically functioning without enough substance, without enough essence. Therefore, the result will be less than positive because their foundation is low or even empty. Imagine trying to produce eggs from your body when the substance it is derived from is depleted. Wouldn't the quality of the eggs be affected if the source that it is deriving its essence from is deficient?

That is why Nutrition plays a large role in the physical condition of the body. Nourishing your body physically with whole foods and their accompanying nutrients is a vital part in your bio-chemistry, assuring that the nutrients needed for organ function and wellbeing are present. Our body uses nutrients for all its processes and if it is lacking in any nutrient then the function of the organ system and of the processes may suffer and not be optimally. When the body is depleted in substance physically and it cannot function, symptoms arise from these imbalances. These symptoms may look like disorders and diseases. The symptoms can be anything from headaches to endometrioses, etc... These symptoms and diseases are the signs telling us the body has an imbalance and something is not functioning correctly.

Therefore, nutrition plays a key role in the well being of our body, along with our mental and emotional health. One way to honor our health, as we mentioned above is to try to eat as close to their natural state as possible, avoiding foods that are processed and altered in any way. The way nature intended food is always the best and ideal for our health. This includes eating organic whenever possible. Organic foods allow us to lessen the chemical content of our foods as well as enhance the quality of the food itself. The soil from organic foods has not been as depleted by the chemical process so it is usually more nutritious than most others.

Continuing on this path includes eating foods with less additives, preservatives, or colors, or added sugar. Also try to eat foods that are cooked naturally, not micro waved, so that the nutrients are better preserved.

Overall, in my years of working with patients I have advocated many forms of eating and types of food for our health. However, I feel that an alkalizing diet provides a quick form of cleansing and allows us to absorb nutrients quickly in our system. Even though I advocate a strong discipline of Alkalizing to quickly establish a healthy state, I also feel strongly that each body is different and that each person needs to determine for themselves and judge for themselves what is best for them.

Alkalizing is therefore a temporary form of eating to make maximum changes of clearing and detoxifying the body in a shortened period of time. Overall, I feel a more balanced system of eating, incorporating a program of balanced foods, such as the hormonal diet is best suited for overall long term health.

It is important to honor our body and take responsibility with our actions. If we, for example, know that caffeine has adverse effects on our energy, depletes our nutrients, plus lowers thyroid, and interferes with fertility, it would be dishonest of ourselves to continue to take it and believe that it would not affect us in this way. Yet on the other hand how much we could have would depend on our inner connection to ourselves, perhaps in our present condition to have a cup of coffee once a week would be okay, versus someone else that may be affected too greatly by having it once a week and their bodies would say none at all for now.

It is hard to admit these things to ourselves because our desire to have it causes us to be in denial and we may feel invincible to the effects of some foods. This is why it is helpful to have a guideline of what to do and eat for optimum health.

I recommend the following: I will write out a list and explain the philosophy behind the recommendations. As you read these things there will be a part of you that will resonate with this information and feel a strong pull to try it, even though it may seem very difficult and you may have to give up foods you enjoy temporarily. I say temporarily because even though I advocate this Alkalizing theory overall, once you have achieved your results then there is more room for flexibility. At the beginning of this process it is best to be as strict as possible and to set clear boundaries.

Making A Nutritional Choice

Again, this process may be a little challenging at first but you have to understand why you are making these choices. One reason is that you would choose to honor your body and create health within that will help you reach your goal of conceiving. Secondly, you want to feel better and eat the foods that will allow your body to function with more energy, more aliveness, and less physiological disorders. Eventually one gets to a point that one is able to accept the changes and is willing to give up the unhealthy foods because you value the long term benefit more than the instant gratification. Once you realize these choices of honoring your body, it then becomes easier to make the decision to be strict because you want to truly take care of your body, rather than because someone is telling you to do so.

If when you read this food information you do not feel a strong pull in your heart to follow it, you may then want to explore the reason why. Does this not feel like an appropriate way of eating for you right now? Is there a way to fine tune this to fit for you? Perhaps you need more protein, or to decrease instead of eliminate something completely? Just be aware that the decision you are making is not from a desire of a food or an addiction to a food choice. Remember that any food choice is just that, food choices. We are so accustomed to thinking that if we don't have a certain type of food we will not be happy.

Food is supposed to supply us with energy and nutrients vital to the physiological functioning of our body. Food is not designed to provide pleasure on a continuous basis. When we are making decisions about what nutrients to eat, try to suspend the pleasure factor for a minute and think of food just as a tool to provide nutrients into our body. This may be a bit challenging. It is not how we are raised and supported in our society, but it is a healthy way to look at our nutrients.

Facts To Be Considered

Attribution to Fertility and Nutrition

Nutrition can have an amazing impact on Fertility. I have seen it over and over again in my office and it is well documented in places around the country. A study conducted at Surrey University in the United Kingdom, revealed that more than 80% of couples with a history of miscarriage or infertility could be helped by changing their diet. All refined foods, alcohol, allergy foods were eliminated and particular attention went to correcting vitamin and mineral deficiencies as well as reducing toxic metal levels. More than 400 couples participated in the study and 81percent conceived, of the 81% who successfully conceived, no babies were born before 36 weeks and none was lighter than 5 pounds 3 ounces!"

According to the internet health library
(http://www.internethealthlibrary.com/Health-problems/Infertility-%20researchDiet&Lifestyle.htma) "It is thought that the endocrine system switches off the reproductive system when the diet is nutritionally deficient. One nutritionist writing in the British Nutrition Foundation Bulletin wrote that the diet before conception plays an important influence on her (the mother's) capacity to bear a healthy child.

In addition, Michael Van Straten, Naturopath and author of Super Foods states: "The nutritional state of women - and of their sexual partners - in the three months before conception is the key to the presence or absence of many birth defects... and reduces the likelihood of infertility." He goes on to recommend that refined carbohydrates (eg. white bread, white rice etc), and coffee, alcohol, meat and all fats must be avoided."

1. Less Protein is Healthier

Less protein equals less accumulation and less out of balance growths such as endometriosis, fibroids, cysts, etc... According to studies, the average American consumes one and a half to four times the amount of protein required by the body consisting of meat, cheese, milk, ice cream, and other products that contain not only protein, but also saturated fat and cholesterol. It has been documented that our bodies contain only 7 percent protein and so much protein can definitely cause imbalances in our overall system.

It is important to note that we do not need to eat the large amounts of protein that we are being told by special interest companies, in order to maintain health. On the contrary, the American Dietetic Association states that a vegetarian diet can provide the sub-cellular units and the amino acids to make protein in amounts that are congruent with the body's needs.

2. Hydration is Important

From my past in working with women in general, I have found that the average woman drinks perhaps three to four cups of water a day. This is an extremely low amount. Even though, people have been made aware to drink at least 8 cups a day of 8 ounces each (64 ounces total), still a busy lifestyle seems to interfere with their ability or desire to do so.

It is very easy to dehydrate our body and create severe biochemical imbalances because of it. We should be drinking not only the 64 ounces usually recommended but actually adding another 64 ounces in order to flush out unwanted toxins on a daily basis.

The recommendation with an Alkalizing program is to drink at least three to four liters a day of good quality water. Distilled or reverse-osmosis (purified) water are more beneficial for the body.

3. Yeast Produces more Yeast and Dampness

Goods made from flour, especially white flour such as bread, muffins, pies, cakes and pastries should be avoided. According to the American Cancer Society, one out of nine American women will develop breast cancer by age 80. Research links it with the ingestion of baked goods and bakers or brewers yeast. Not only may there be a correlation with Cancer, but it also creates the condition of "dampness" or "yeast/candida" in the body, which are commonly documented with patients having Infertility related conditions.

4. Diary Contributes to Acidifying Of the Body

Dairy products create acidity in the body and accumulate as well. These products also contain the presence of yeast and fungus, molds, and their by-products, which certainly are detrimental to the biochemistry within. Also, due to the high sugar and fat content of dairy products, the fact that dairy cows are fed stored grains and fungal-based antibiotics, and the fermentation process of cheese and yogurt, all dairy products should be eventually eliminated from the

171

diet. Calcium can be obtained from green leafy vegetables, green drinks, calcium-fortified tofu and soymilk, collards, broccoli, okra, salmon, etc.

A report by M. Kushi, author, explains some of the detrimental correlations with diary and the reproductive system. "Casein, the protein in cheese, milk, cream, butter, and other dairy foods cannot be assimilated easily and begins to accumulate in an undigested state in the upper intestine, putrefying, producing toxins, and leading to a weakening of the gastric, intestinal, pancreatic, and biliary systems, as well as mucous deposits. The inability to digest milk or other dairy products is known as lactose intolerance and is found in about 50 to 90 percent of the world's population groups with the exception of those of Scandinavian origin and some other European ancestries." He continues, "Dairy food affects all the organs and systems. However, because it is a product of the mammary gland, it primarily affects the human glands and related structures, especially the reproductive organs. The most commonly affected are the breasts, uterus, ovaries, prostate, thyroid, nasal cavities, pituitary gland, the cochlea in the ear, and the cerebral area surrounding the midbrain. Its adverse effects first appear as the accumulation of mucus and fat and then the formation of cysts, tumors, and finally cancer. Many people who eat dairy food have mucous accumulations in the nasal cavities and inner ear, resulting in hay fever and hearing difficulty. Accumulation of fatty deposits from dairy food in the kidneys and also gallbladder leads to stones."

"The development of breast cysts, breast tumors, and finally breast cancer follows a similar pattern. Common problems from dairy, in combination with other factors, are vaginal discharges, ovarian cysts, fibrosis and uterine cancer, ovarian cancer, and prostate fat accumulation with cyst formation. Many diseases of the reproductive organs, including infertility, are associated with dairy consumption."

Source; Mishio Kushi from
http://home.iae.nl/users/lightnet/health/meat.htm

5. Alcohol can Lower Your Conception Chances

Wine, beer, whiskey, brandy, gin, rum and vodka are purely mycotoxic. Alcohol is a fungus-produced mycotoxin made by yeast that causes direct injury to human health. Through a study by the Washington University School of Medicine, Science News Vol. 146, it has been shown that the use of alcohol reduces fertility by 50 percent.

6. Smoking Ages the Ovaries

Tobacco leaves are coated with yeast, fungus, and mycotoxins, which poison the cells and tissues of the body. Research clearly reveals the pathway that the fermentation of the tobacco creates with yeast and sugar. When using tobacco, you are directly introducing dried fungus and wastes into your body. Furthermore, nicotine ages the ovaries and makes the eggs resistant to fertilization.

7. Quit the Coffee

Not only is it acidic but there is some pretty interesting studies on how coffee contributes to infertility. In a study by (1990) Yale University School of Medicine, Drs. Larry Dulgosz and Michael B. Brachs concluded that women were at an elevated risk of Infertility of 55 percent greater, if they drank one cup of coffee. They had a 100 percent greater chance or infertility if they drank one and ½ cups of coffee and 176 percent higher for women drinking three cups of coffee per day.

Also, coffee drinking before and during pregnancy was associated with more than twice the risk of miscarriage when the mother consumed two to three cups of coffee per day. This was sited by Dr. Claire Infante-Rivard of the Dept. of Occupation Health at McGill University, Quebec Canada, Journal of the American Medical Association, 1993.

8. Beware of the MSG and other Food Additives: Eat Organic

MSG, monosodium glutamate, which is a common flavor enhancer added in foods, was found to cause infertility problems of various kinds including reduced success rates by 50 percent. MSG is found in *ACCENT,* flavored potato chips, Doritos, Cheetos, meat seasonings and many packaged soups. Studies done by Drs. William J. Pizzi, June E. Barnhart, et. al. Dept. of Psychology, Northeastern Illinois University, Chicago, 1979.

Furthermore, it is clearly important to eat organic whenever possible, avoiding all unnecessary and potentially dangerous additives that only serve to intoxicate and deteriorate your health.

9. Beware of Environment Estrogens

Environmental estrogens are chemicals which "mimic" our natural estrogens and which may be interfering with the delicate balance of natural estrogens that are necessary for reproductive success, according to Dr. Susan Jobling, Tracey Reynolds, Roger White, Malcolm G. Parker, and John Sumpter at the Dept. of Biology and Biochemistry, at Brunel University, London 1995. They state "A proper balance of natural estrogens in the body is essential for reproductive success. However, reports have been suggesting that

175

environmental estrogens (chemicals which "mimic" our natural estrogens) are creating infertility problems by confusing the body's estrogen receptors. Some pesticides have already been shown to be environmental estrogens. New research shows that more chemicals are being found to be environmental estrogens including the food additives butylated hydroxyanisole (BHA) Other chemicals found to be somewhat estrogenic include, PVC plastics."

http://www.chemtox.com/infertility/download/InfertilityFacts.pdf

Alkalizing

The Alkaline theory is based on using alkaline foods to maintain the pH level of our blood balanced. When the pH level is unbalanced it affects the blood which in turn affects all organ systems in our body. It affects our heart, our nervous system, our lymphatic system, and even our reproductive system. Therefore, a great indicator of your general health is your pH level, or how acidic or alkaline your body environment is. The scale starts at 1.0 (acid) to 14.0 (alkaline) with 7.0 being neutral. It is important for the blood to be at a neutral level for survival and your body will fight to function at this level.

The problem begins when we eat the foods that we are accustomed to such as simple carbohydrates and even whole carbohydrates, meats, diary products, sugars, etc… All these foods are acidic. When we eat very little vegetables, which are alkaline, we are giving our bodies an over abundance of acidic foods, which create an acidic environment which it has to balance on its own.

When the body has an acidic environment, it is the perfect home for yeast, fungi, mold bacteria, viruses, and the like (known as microforms). This is why an acidic environment can be conducive to problems such as yeast infections and other types of damp type accumulations affecting the reproductive system.

So, overall the over acidification of our bodies create the perfect internal environment for toxicity formed by these microforms and can easily contribute to stagnation and dampness disorders within our reproductive system. This over acidification can be greatly corrected by eating a balance of alkalizing foods versus an excess of acidic foods.

It is important to note that over acidic blood taxes the immune system in an attempt to carry out the acid, so that it can function at the necessary balanced level of (7.365). This taxation on the immune system can lead to all sorts of responses with immune issues in fertility, contributing to antibodies affecting negatively sperm and embryos.

The good news is that you have a lot of control with what you eat and can create health through your food choices. For further detail on the alkalizing theory, a great source is the PH Miracle by Robert O. Young 2002. He has been developing this theory for quite a few years, with much success in various areas of health.

Alkaline food and water must be consumed in order to provide the needed nutrients for the body to neutralize acids and toxins in the blood, lymph, and tissues, while strengthening immune function and organ systems. For this reason, the Alkalarian Diet was developed to guide those who wish to regain balance and vigor in the body. Some people may choose to follow the Alkalarian Diet completely, while others slowly transition themselves and their family. For many, the change is not an overnight event, but a process. Taste buds that have been jaded by the toxic effect of sugar, salt, and other artificial flavors may take some time to adjust and appreciate the subtler taste of whole foods.

In general, 70% to 80% of your foods should come from fresh vegetables, grasses, sprouts, low – sugar fruits and good fats (especially avocado and coconut). Try to eat as much raw foods as possible, but cooked and steamed is good. Use olive oil specifically to cook with. Choosing a variety of vegetables with most of them green, allows you to eat a good source of alkaline food that will help to balance the excess acids in the blood.

The remaining 20%-30% of your food should be fish, nuts and seeds and whole grains that are less acidic; millet, buckwheat and spelt. Although rice and wheat are whole grains, they are higher in acids, therefore not as recommended to be eaten as often. In this 20% of your food you may also add mildly acidic foods such as potatoes or preferably sweet potato.

I do want to add that even though eating red meat is not in line with alkalizing, I have seen many cases of women that need to have red meat in their system, and for this I advocate a high quality of red meat, free from hormones or chemicals, to be ingested preferably once to twice a week. Drink plenty of water with a Greens powder in them. At least starting with two liters and working your way up to three liters three a day.

What are Green Powders?

Green Powders are alkalizing powders made from green vegetables, grasses, sprouted grains that contain vitamins to and nutrients that you would not likely be consumed on a daily basis. There are many good ones on the market, the best way choose is to make sure that they contain no sea vegetables or algae, and that they do contain mainly vegetables with very little fruits or grains. Organic greens are better of course for your body. More than a pound of produce is required to make just 1 ounce of green powders.

Drinking greens in your water on a daily basis helps your body to detoxify and nourish the cells for healthier quality, which in turn nourishes all the organ systems, including the reproductive system.

Where to Begin

It is helpful to make some changes slowly and integrate them well into your everyday life. If, of course time is an issue, i.e.; you are close to 40 years old and would like to make some fast severe changes in your system, then a more aggressive approach is required.

I recommend all my patients to make at least one change a week, depending on the degree of those changes, but I do not advocate making two and three severe changes in the same week. For example, for a person that is a heavy coffee drinker and eats plenty of dairy, as well as an avid consumer of red meat and fast food, I would recommend first eliminating the fast food and one other type of food group, such as dairy. After about a week's time, I would incorporate other changes for that person, so that the body has time to adapt and assimilate the changes. But on the other hand, if a patient only ate some dairy with a small amount of two or three other undesirable food groups in their diet, I would then recommend the elimination of more than one food group from their diet at a time.

After you read the list, determine what changes you want to make without becoming overwhelmed. Below is a list of foods that are acidic in nature and are best eliminated completely.

Eliminate

Sugar (simple sugars) sugar, sweeteners, sugar in any form.

White flour

Wheat (limit to once a week)

Processed frozen or fast foods

Alcohol

Caffeine

Sodas

Any foods with Preservatives, color or additives

Butter (replace with olive oil)

Diary

Red Meat (or lessen the frequency)

Chicken (limit quantity)

Turkey (limit quantity)

Fruits (high in sugar – limit quantity)

Increase

Vegetables (organic and leafy green)

Whole grains (brown rice, millet, oatmeal, barley, spelt)

Soy protein (only if there is not low thyroid issues)

Fish

Eggs

Beans

Almonds and Nuts

Water (good quality)

The indications above show you a general idea of what the overall alkalizing program looks like. Your foods will mainly come from these categories above in the 70%-30% ratio mentioned above. Below we have adapted a complete list of foods to shop for from the "Back to the House of Health" by Shelley Young 1999.

Food List

Seeds	Flax	Pumpkin
Sunflower	Sesame	

Nuts	Almonds	Hazelnuts
Pecans	Pine Nuts	Brazil Nuts
Macademia		

Grains	Millet	Kamut
Quinoa	Amaranth	

Adzuki	Lentils	Pinto
Kidney	Mung	Garbanzo
Black	Black- Eyed	

Fresh Vegetables		
Baby Greens	Zucchini	Cauliflower
Larger leafy greens	Sprouts	Broccoli
Spinach	Radishes	Beets
Kale	Onions	Cabbage
Chili Peppers	Celery	Squash
Avocado	Parsley	Tomato
Carrots	Peppers	Cucumber
	Fruits	

Lemon	Lime	White
Grapefruit	Blueberries	Raspberries

Other Items	
Rice Milk (Make sure it does not have cane syrup) (No sugar added)	Almond Milk
Hummus	Almond Butter
Roasted Bell peppers packed in oil	Vegetable Broth
Oils (Olive, Flax seed, Udo's choice blend)	Tahini

Gradual Process

If this sounds a little mind boggling I will try to simplify it for you. Here are other guidelines to simplify your process:

Eat mainly green vegetables for 70%-80% percent of your diet and 20%-30% percent of cooked, warmed or mildly acidifying foods.

Recommendations to start:
1. Cut out all foods not on above shopping list.
2. Eat a salad or vegetables with each meal.
3. Reduce meat and increase fish at least in one meal a day.
4. Eliminate all flour products and sugars from your diet.
5. Drink 2-3 liters of super greens a day to begin.

Food Combining

Food combining is another part of this program because it allows foods to be digested appropriately, avoiding mycotoxins and growth in our blood streams.

In order to combine foods properly the following should be adhered to.
1. Eat grains, starches only with vegetables; do not combine proteins with grains in the same meal.

2. Eat proteins only with vegetables; do not combine grains or starches with protein in the same meal.

3. Eating fruits should be done by itself. You should wait approximately 2 hours before you have any other food after your fruits. Please remember that most fruits are not alkalizing, so they should not be on your program. Adhere to only lemons, limes, and white grapefruit.

Monitoring Progress

With reproductive issues it may become a little difficult to monitor immediate progress because it takes approximate 30 days for a complete cycle, and for changes to be noticed in the cycle itself. Nonetheless, you may see other changes and improvements in many of the following areas.

Physical Changes

It is easier to see the changes if there are a lot of symptoms to begin with. If you experience headaches on a daily basis, have no energy and have heartburn every day, it is easy to notice when these things start improving. On the other hand, physical changes may be subtle; you may notice a sounder sleep and slightly more energy upon waking up.

Please remember that your body has to make huge changes

internally before you actually notice them on a physical level. Many changes have to take place on organ systems, before they are noticeable physically. So I caution patience is of utmost importance.

For example, I had a patient that spotted for 15 days out of the month, had very irregular periods and severe backaches. She began improving with a couple days less of spotting for the first two months, then her periods started coming on the same day every month. After about six months there was no more spotting and her periods were regular and her backaches diminished by at least 80%. As she continued to work with me and support her new changes she became pregnant in her ninth month of treatment. And now has a healthy baby girl.

This is not to say that progress is always slow, but it is important to point out that the body takes time to adjust to the new information and integrate nutrients it is being given, fill in the gaps and function from a new place. You are not using a "drug" that forces changes immediately and is forcing the body function differently, even if temporarily. You are changing the foundation of how your body works, and how it has been working for years and years, perhaps even for your whole life. And that takes time.

Emotional Changes

Emotional changes are very important with this type of work. It is common to hear people say that they feel more "relaxed, more centered, less anxious". This is a very common response to healing. Many times the emotional changes are noticeable before the physical changes, even more so if there are few physical symptoms.

In fertility cases, the progress may be slow and this may test your patience. However, it is important to have the focus on healing your whole body/mind and bringing you closer in connection with your spirit. The focus is that you are truly centering on what nourishes your complete Self and this alone will bring you great joy, not just from a possible pregnancy, but from a bigger picture of health and joy into your own being and your life.

This type of focus helps you to be gentle and patient with yourself, so that your expectations do not ruin your progress. It also helps to understand that it is a process rather than a magic pill. The magic is in the process and the only way to the other side is through it, putting in the time and focus on yourself.

Which Fish is Safe?

According to the National Resources Defense Council the safest fish to eat according to the levels of toxic mercury listed below:

Least Mercury
Anchovies
Butterfish
Catfish
Clam
Crab (Domestic)
Crawfish/Crayfish
Croaker (Atlantic)
Flounder
Haddock (Atlantic)
Hake
Herring
Mackerel (N. Atlantic, Chub)
Mullet
Oyster
Perch (Ocean)
Plaice
Pollock
Salmon (Canned)
Salmon (Fresh)
Sardine
Scallop
Shad (American)
Shrimp
Sole (Pacific)
Squid (Calamari)
Tilapia
Trout (Freshwater)
Whitefish
Whiting

Moderate Mercury
Eat six servings or less per month:
Bass (Striped, Black)
Carp
Cod (Alaskan)
Croaker (White Pacific)
Halibut (Atlantic)
Halibut (Pacific)
Jacksmelt
(Silverside)
Lobster
Mahi Mahi
Monkfish
Perch (Freshwater)
Sablefish
Skate
Snapper
Tuna (Canned chunk light)
Tuna (Skipjack)
Weakfish (Sea Trout)

High Mercury	**Highest Mercury**
Eat three servings or less per month:	*Avoid eating:*
	Mackerel (King)
Bluefish	Marlin
Grouper	Orange Roughy
Mackerel (Spanish, Gulf)	Shark
Sea Bass (Chilean)	Swordfish
Tuna (Canned Albacore)	Tilefish
Tuna (Yellowfin)	Tuna (Bigeye, Ahi)

Sample Menu

These sample menus can help put the foods into perspective. Be aware that the foods below can be interchanged, especially lunch and dinner. The important things are to keep most food choices to 70-80% percent alkaline foods (mainly vegetables and 20-30% of proteins or complex carbohydrates (either one or the other, not both in one meal). Breakfast choices tend to be more lenient of that 70-30 ratio but that is a personal choice.

BREAKFAST:

Sprouted Grain toast with Soy Milk, almond or rice milk.
Or
Multi grain cereal (with no sugar) with soy, almond or rice milk.
Or
Avocadoes and tomatoes.
Or

Spinach with eggs.
Or
Grapefruit with eggs.
Or
Oatmeal with raisins.

LUNCH:

Salad/ Avocado
Or
Salad/ Beans
Or
Vegetable Soup with Brown Rice
Or
Salad & Vegetable Roll Up with Sprouted Bread.

DINNER:

Salad/ Avocado/ and Fish
Or
Salad/ Vegetable Soup/ Fish
Or
Stir Fry Vegetables with Tofu or any other protein
Or
Salad/ Brown Rice/ Steam vegetables
Or
Roasted Vegetables/ Bean soup

Use snacks such as almonds and fruits, such as almonds, blueberries, raspberries, blackberries, strawberries, apples, grapefruit, in between meals.

Environmental Hazards

It is not only important to eat organically, but in order to maintain the health of our body it is important to decrease the toxicity levels. Studies have showed that our reproductive systems are affected by toxins in our environment and that we ingest. Toxins are acidic and cause the destruction of health; this is why staying alkalized is helpful to creating health.

There are many harmful hazards in our environment, in our foods, in our air, water, soil, and even personalities. Even though chemicals, toxins, and pesticides are all around us there are some things we can do to become aware and make healthier choices for ourselves.

Other Helpful Hints

When we look at pesticides in our foods we know that is well documented that they cause health problems and serious damage to the male and female reproductive system. The best way to avoid this is to eat organic foods, foods that are cultivated and grown without harmful chemicals and pesticides. Some of the major chemicals linked with causing harm to our reproductive system are; kepone, DBCP ethylene dibromide, DDT, Chlordane and MSG additive to food.

By avoiding these chemicals and pesticides and eating organically, your body has a higher chance of healing and regaining health.

The other chemicals that are worth mentioning are the chemicals we use on our skin daily. Products such as soaps, shampoos, make-up, skin lotions, perfumes, etc.... can be hazardous to our health, even though they have not been banned in the United States. Phthalates in products have been found to have devastating effects on both men and women's health. Medical disorders such as low sperm count and severe damage in the reproductive systems have been documented with this product, but yet to be banned here. One major challenge is that products are not listed on many perfumes or cosmetics, which is where this chemical is mostly found.

Another chemical that is toxic and harmful is the use of parabens, for example which are estrogen disrupters. Estrogen disrupters are chemicals that can cause your genes to mutate and change as well as imitating other hormones in your body. In essence what this does is create havoc with your body's natural hormones effecting FSH, estrogen and other fine delicate hormonal balances that are crucial to reproduction.

It sounds overwhelming to start to really see what these chemicals are doing to our bodies and the fact that we have to take a stance and make choices to create health in our being. By consciously choosing to eat organically, choosing personal care products that are free from harmful chemicals, and minimizing your exposure to pesticides you can regain balance in this area. Below is a list of products that I have found reputable throughout the years for your use. You may also look up products in the Green Guide, which is usually sold in Health Food Stores. Start to try some of these new sources and products and watch your health increase.

Lotions:
www.Perfectorganics.com
www.Burtsbees.com
www.Origins.com
www.Aubrey-organics.com

Hair:
www.tomsofmaine.com
www.Avalonorganics.com

Soaps:
www.DrBronner.com

CHAPTER 7

Nourishing our Spiritual Body

Deep Within Our Womb

Why is there a rise in infertility in the last 10 years? As women grow stronger on the outside, something seems to be growing weaker on the inside, could our infertility have any correlation to the image of ourselves outside in the world and the roles we play. Perhaps we have had to hide and remold ourselves to fit into our male dominated society, leaving behind essential elements that are crucial to our health, our wellbeing and most importantly our wholeness.

It seems to me that throughout these past decades, as women have grown into a stronger, acceptable image in the outer world, we have subtlety left behind the very aspects of ourselves that we now seek; nurturing, loving, sensitivity and mothering. Can it be that we have displaced these feelings within ourselves in order to survive within the greater demands of our society and consequently shut down our ability to access these qualities when we need them the most; at the time of conception.

And this is not only a phenomenon with infertility but it seems to be common among all gynecological disorders; endometriosis, polycystic ovaries, hormonal imbalances, etc... Our need to be accepted by the larger whole of society has created this subtle sacrifice of parts identified with being feminine. These parts of us that have been judged as weak and somehow defective throughout out centuries have greatly influenced our own acceptance of ourselves. The result is a sense of having to hide these traits of being feminine and somehow appear to compete in the male-dominated world with male accepted qualities; i.e. strength, emotional detachment, less compassion. We have subtlety incorporated the belief that in order to survive, to achieve, to be successful, to be loved and honored, we have to be a certain way, and somehow our own feminine feelings - compassion, nurturing, tenderness, etc., are not accepted. And displaying these certainly is in conflict with achieving the CEO position, or becoming the new vice president.

As women, we have taken on these beliefs and short changed ourselves. We have chosen to become tough, successful, climb the corporate ladder and mold ourselves into women excluding our sensitive, nurturing, and compassionate nature. I am suggesting that we take a look at these part of ourselves that we have had to bury deep within ourselves in order to survive. We can be successful in the outer world and bring all of our self to the table, rather than adapt ourselves to the hard, non-sensitive, non-feminine view. I suggest that to the degree that we compromise who we are is the degree that we have compromised our inner being and created disease and distortion in our bodies.

Now, we are not assuming that every woman has to be overly emotional, or extremely sensitive, but I am suggesting that these traits are not inherently "bad", they are useful and valuable in their own right. And secondly, I am not suggesting that this is the only issue with Infertility, there are many, this is one of the prominent psycho-spiritual dynamics that comes to light with most of the women that I see in practice.

Women carry their history in their DNA, all our emotional, physiological, mental and spiritual history, from family generations through generations. Women have endured so much throughout history, all of this is stored within our cells. Deep inside our womb we hold the very essence of life itself. Sometimes we feel disconnected from our own source of life and instead have replaced it with fear, doubt and terror. These stored feelings are not just from ourselves, but from all the women that have come before us and all our past generations as well as all the future generations. Our womb is our sacredness, as well as our place of pain.

When we experience fertility issues, we are forced to look deep within and open this place up, not just in the physical sense with physical invasion of fertility treatment protocols, but we are forced to question our own abilities to be a mother, to produce, to create offspring, as well as what it means to be a woman. Many of us are confused about what it means to be a woman; we have swung the pendulum from one extreme to the other; from past matriartical societies to complete loss of power and humiliation, to conditional positions of power in the last few decades. But this is on the outside, on the inside there is still much turmoil and pain handed down from the ages, and still the reflection of a silent fight for our rights, for our truth, for our value and to be seen, heard and accepted without having to become something that we are not.

We carry within us the struggle to be seen for who we truly are, not equal necessarily, but that of possessing a special quality of mothering, of caring, and of nurturing that may be different than that of men. There is a yearning within us to become mothers on the outside, and yet we are not able to honor our feminine qualities of motherhood on the inside. We have dishonored and let this part of us die inside, by acting strong, by competing and trying to be the same as men, in our own desperation for recognition, for love and acceptance. We have fought by male rules, instead of creating and honoring our own rules, we have become equal to men, leaving

behind the very same quality we seek and desire in becoming a
mother. We have left behind our ability to mother, to nurture, to be
sensitive, to be soft and perhaps a little less strong than our male
counter parts. Maybe they have the physical strength and perhaps
we have the emotional strength. These traits have been seen as a
weakness in our western culture, so we have chosen to believe in our
inherent weaknesses and then continue to try to prove that we were
not weak, by denying this part of our essence.

Over the years women have felt helpless, wrong, fearful, and weak
and in many ways have found powerful jobs, became "independent",
become tougher, done more, sought more control, all in order to
compensate for that dark place within that keeps making us feel
invalid. It is not that we cannot have these powerful jobs, or become
independent, but seeking it in order to comfort our inner levels of
insecurity and void leaves us feeling our inner levels of insecurity
and void, it will never complete us. We continue to try harder
outside, while inside the void gets bigger and bigger, the pain gets
bigger and bigger and our despair grows along with our disease.

As women desiring to carry our place in the fabric of society, we
have unequally been judged and been measured by a standard that
does not allow our essence to be. By trying to be equal to our male
counterparts, rather than honoring our special gifts and differences,

199

we have denied an essential part of ourselves that provides the special traits of motherhood itself.

Perhaps we haven't completely compromised our being, but just by being a woman in this society, we carry the seed of the history of this pain in the mass group consciousness because it is part of our societal environment and the unwritten rules that we play by in our western world. The unspoken and sometimes spoken judgments of our feminine qualities are an ingrained part of our psyche and the road that women have been walking through for quite some time.

Deep within our wombs, we hold deep seated feelings of being a woman. We hold all the negative feelings that do not fit with our western culture's view and our own view (by default) of what women "should" be. These beliefs include thoughts that we are weak, we are too sensitive, we shouldn't cry, we talk too much, worry too much, we are not competent enough, we are not strong enough, we are not strict enough, we have too many feelings, we have too much fear, etc… Which ones did you take on about yourself? Essentially, we have felt that we don't measure up and all the aspects of ourselves that don't measure up, we store, hide and disown, and many times within our wombs.

As women, we are different from men, generally we have different qualities. This does not take away from our importance in the fabric of life, it actually adds to it. We play an important role and one of them is motherhood. One way of deeply healing our wombs is by exploring our deeper beliefs and feelings around being a woman, around mother hood, what we hate about being female, what we feel bad about within ourselves and what we have disowned in an erroneous attempt to survive and be accepted in our culture.

It is time we own all of ourselves and honored ourselves as women, complete with all the aspects that we "dislike" and that make us seem "weak". These are the very qualities we are in need of embracing to become mothers and step into our true womanhood. The good news is that we are only responsible for our part in it. As we change our own beliefs and accept all the disowned aspects of ourselves, we heal ourselves, one by one, and our society at large.

In order to explore our deep seated belief of the feminine quality within the matrix of our wombs, it is important to build our trust and connection to our wholeness, our divine essence. It is important to tap into your beliefs around our Divine nature, the source within us, that is benign and that has a divine level of organization and purpose. Perhaps it is helpful to think of this source as having a higher purpose for our wellbeing. Nonetheless, no matter how we think of our higher source, it is real, it is always part of us, no matter how disconnected we feel from it. It is important to have our divine essence as a focal point within ourselves.

Our connection point to our Divine essence can begin in our heart, this is an entry point to our divine source, a higher source that has our best interest at heart, even though we may not understand or see how the current events are manifesting accordance to that truth. But nonetheless, as we start to move towards this light within, we start to discharge all the beliefs that are not aligned with our divine essence of who we are. We are then able to begin to connect with our hearts and our divine female qualities in our wombs. We are then able to allow this essence to wash over all the painful misconceptions, beliefs and thoughts that we have carried throughout our existence. As we do this we begin the healing of our minds and emotions, as well as physical body and our spiritual selves.

This place deep inside our wombs is hungry for the nourishment of pure divine essence. Reproductive disorders and infertility disorders are viewed as issues of "essence" in Traditional Chinese Medicine (TCM). In TCM "essence" is what is carried in the male and female in order to create life. From a spiritual viewpoint, essence is the source that feeds us, a divine spiritual essence. And from my experience many that are suffering with fertility issues are suffering from a disconnection from their very own essence, a lack of conscious awareness of their divine essence and qualities that they inherently carry within their female forms. Instead, they are functioning from the painful history that women have reduced themselves to believe and consequently the physical form shows all the distortions of such limited consciousness.

Many alternative treatments nourish this essence greatly and start to reestablish our awareness of our divine essence, whether it is through breathing, meditation, visualization, acupuncture, aromatherapy, herbal therapies or spiritual healings. Each discipline may do it slightly different, but each with a specific strand that helps to establish the wholeness and create health.

Embracing the Wholeness of the Feminine

The woman holds all the treasures of creation deep within her being, and to know herself is to know the truth of what she carries. This treasure within the female creation is the essence of life; it is the manifestation of all that is. This divine essence that is at the core of who we are is like the essence of the Earth, a deep well for life itself to spring forth from. We are the earth, we are that essence that carries all the qualities of the Divine; love, peace, beauty, freedom, caring, compassion, mothering, gentleness, intuitiveness, strength and knowing, to name a few. To know this truth about the feminine within us, is to allow ourselves the freedom to be who we are, without identifying our self worth with the outer experiences or with the state of health in our body. In other words, it is possible for our body to manifest disorders and still have an understanding that we are whole within. What we are and what we carry is a very deep truth of the wholeness, regardless of our awareness of it and current manifestation physically.

Therefore, if we are incapable of seeing our own inner beauty and seeing that we are made with indescribable beauty within, then we may only see and believe what society and our outer world says is beauty and how their limited definition of it. If we do not know and believe that we carry the peace and strength, but rather judge ourselves as weak and overly emotional, for example, then we will make our emotions wrong, and our intuition wrong, and identify only with society's limited view of what strength is.

Our society holds a male/dominant perspective view that in general does not honor women and their gifts and their true nature. (For a more complete history on societal views on the feminine throughout the existence of time, read Raine Eisler's "The Chalice and the Blade"). Nonetheless, it is important for us to understand what the feminine creation is and all that we carry within ourselves. Our strength may not be in outer physical strength, but it is nonetheless just as powerful in a more subtle way. The strength of the feminine creation is in upholding truth, being in alignment with our deeper values, with the divine essence, being in alignment with creation, and allowing creation to pour through us and create abundantly. Our strength is in being a vessel for the spirit of Earth itself to manifest... whether it is in a new project, in a career, a baby, a home or any vessel that pours love and gives to everyone. Our strength is in our ability to care, to love, to show compassion, to know what someone needs, to mother, to nurture, to contain, to love unconditionally and to give, knowing that there is an endless source that we are connected to that never stops giving. These are different qualities than outer physical strength, but both have their own value. We don't have to have outer strength to be strong; but rather value our own sense of strength.

Our worthiness is one of the biggest spiritual obstacles that stand in the way regarding issues of fertility. Our fertility issues are connected with the ability to honor who we are as women and transform the negative pictures that we have invested ourselves in, to the highest belief that truly honors who we are. As we explore our thoughts, beliefs and feelings about who we are and who we think we are, we have to be willing to cross these barriers to the other side. As women we give birth to the creation and we traditionally nurture the creation in one way or another. In order to allow ourselves to do this, which involves conceiving, we have to believe that we are worth carrying this responsibility and that we are capable and worthy to do so.

Just like any disease, at the spiritual level, Infertility becomes about transformation of a virtue... from unworthiness to worthiness, as well as love, essence, peace, truth and value. It is about accepting that we are worthy of having the highest honor of being the vessel that brings life into creation, and continues life on this planet. And this process involves letting go of all the other pictures of who we think we are, and what we think is wrong with us.

Deep within our being we hold a divine essence which has been described by a mystic Sufi master as "a jewel". This jewel is the deep essence within us that we carry our divine light in form of the divine qualities, and especially of the Feminine. These qualities are peace, beauty, compassion, gentleness, creativity, deep potential, truth, patience, deep acceptance, deep forgiveness, and many, many more. By beginning to embrace these within ourselves, we are able to transform all aspects of our lives and our consciousness, including our diseases. This wholeness is true healing, to be able to touch this place within, changes our relationship with ourselves, and allows us to be and express who we truly are. We do not need to become whole, but rather wash away all the layers that we have created in our humanity, that cover up our wholeness. We are already whole.

Acceptance in Our Being and the World Around Us

Acceptance is a place deep within us that opens many doors. It opens the door of choices, it opens the door of peace, and it opens the door to change. It may be hard to imagine that accepting something actually allows it to change. How can that be, we ask ourselves? In my understanding, when we accept things we are seeing them for what they are, possibly acknowledging that there is a higher order at play, letting it have the space and room that it needs to exist and not resisting it. In this way, there is no denial of the trait or situation, therefore, it doesn't persist. It has true space to be and be released or transformed into a higher vibration.

When we can't accept something, we quickly try to change it, our minds try to figure something out in order to fix it, to repair the situation, make it better but at the same time avoiding the original event or situation.

Deep acceptance allows us to really see and perhaps even come to terms with the facts as they are. It is like taking a pause when things aren't what you want them to be. It's not trying to figure it out, or jumping to solve it, just pausing with an acknowledgement that this is where you are at, even if you don't like it. And to add to that, we can accept that even though you don't like where things are at, in this moment, there is a higher order, an conscious intelligence at play and we may rest on that knowing. We can rest on the knowing that we can trust that there is a reason, a conscious order, so that it is not absolutely up to us alone, and we are not alone in making everything work "right".

From that perspective, we can start to become free to take action, from a place that we know we are supported by the divine order of things, by the consciousness of light in the Universe. And when we make choices from this place, there is much more ease and peace with every move, rather than falling back into our pain. Most people fear accepting their circumstances because they think it means having to resign to how things are and believe that they will continue this way forever. But in fact, you are just acknowledging the way things are at the moment, rather than a denial of them, and also acknowledging your own desire for them to change and to be different. Acceptance can mean to accept that, for example, you have not been able to conceive in the last two years, and that you also have a deep desire to conceive and have a baby. Acceptance may also mean acknowledging your feelings around this situation and the difficulty it has presented you with, as well as the pain and suffering you have experienced around it.

When we have a situation that is difficult for us, for example, recurring miscarriages; it is difficult to accept it and easy to just want to avoid it or fix it. But that doesn't always work and usually prolongs the pain deeply in our being, and we suffer greatly because of it. Then, when we become pregnant again, we are prone to re-experience the fear of the previous miscarriage and the suffering because we really haven't completely let go of that suffering within us. That pain is still there and we are avoiding it because it may feel overwhelmingly painful for us to face.

Hence, it is important to accept our situation, our defeats, and our issues with fertility even if we want to avoid the pain and the disappointment. And as a reminder, in order to change the physiology underlining the fertility issue it is important to face these places within ourselves. Accepting them is part of feeling that you may be feeling sad, disappointed, confused and helpless at your experience of infertility. And yet you can start to acknowledge that even in that pain, there is a higher order of consciousness that can heal this pain if you allow this conscious light to come in and heal these places of pain. Even if you don't understand why this is happening to you, you don't have to figure it all out, before you can receive healing around it.

Once you have accepted these situations and conditions in the present moment, and given yourself some time with your feelings, know that you do have choices and you can choose what you will do next. You can choose to do nothing and take a break or explore alternative medicine, pursue western treatments, consider adoption, reevaluate your choices of becoming a parent, or consider reflection and inner healing. There are many choices, and your mind and sometimes the authorities in the field; i.e. doctors, etc., will give you a limited option of choices and this is only because of their limited awareness. Nonetheless, you are truly freer to choose when you have accepted a difficult situation and acknowledged a conscious presence within it and within yourself at which is present at all times.

Accepting What Is

When we are connected to our spiritual source we have a little more trust, a little more acceptance and we are able to look at the big picture and what that may be bringing to our plate. In other words, there are things that we can not control, probably most things in this life. And when we have a solid place of trust within us, we are able to look at these events in our life with a little more compassion towards ourselves and a little less expectation of what we need to have in order to fulfill our needs.

When we accept what is we are able to see the gifts inherent in a painful situation, even if not immediately, but perhaps with time. Accepting the possibility that there is a divine order within every situation and that instead of stopping with the pain of the situation, we can open ourselves to see a deeper truth and blessing inherent an otherwise seemingly painful situation.

Releasing the Old Pictures, Receiving the Healing and Connecting With the Jewel

As Women we are part of the Divine creation, made with a body that is sacred and holy in many ways. The "Jewel" within is the essence of this connection we all have to the divine, male and female, it is our wholeness. This jewel in our hearts, as it is referred to by many spiritual paths and it connects us to the consciousness of light in our deep heart, from which all healing emanates. This is also our well of wholeness and the place where we are complete. From this consciousness of light, all our pictures of how we saw ourselves, as well as how we think about ourselves can be washed and brought back into truth and wholeness. Through our deep connection in our hearts, we can wash away our pain and suffering and all the erroneous beliefs that we have created from our humanity.

This wholeness consciousness that we carry deep in our hearts is the place where we carry the beautiful qualities of the light. These are qualities that we all yearn for such as joy, happiness, peace, mercy, love, justice, truth and patience. These qualities are said to be the qualities of the Divine Essence and the essential truth of life. When we allow these Light qualities to fill our heart and soul, they also start to transform all the deeply held beliefs that we have acquired in our minds, emotions and physical body. As this light consciousness expands, our focus turns towards these qualities and we are able to experience more of these qualities in our lives, filling the places of unworthiness and emptiness and transforming the other negative qualities such as fear, despair, disappointment, anger, rage, and many more.

True healing occurs in our hearts and in our beings with these qualities of light, and miraculously our pain and suffering is overridden by their bounty. Our life and our experiences begin to change and the internal and external dance of attraction starts to change our world inside and outside. Our physical bodies start to heal on all levels just by the acceptance of returning ourselves to our wholeness within and discovering our Jewel.

As our emotions and mind start to feel better, our physical body also starts to respond by returning to a healthier state. Our biology returns to a natural state of health and wellbeing, which is the true healing in the body. Once the bio-chemistry and the functioning of the organ systems start to be effected, healing moves through the physical dimension and is seen in the correction of physical disorders.

Patients with polycystic ovaries become pregnant, women with histories of miscarriages can now hold a baby full term, and endometriosis doesn't stop other women from conceiving. Women with unexplained infertility become pregnant after five years of trying, and even more miraculously women with failed IVFs that dared to hope and persevere, become pregnant.

So how do we get to this point, you may be asking yourself. How do we connect with this consciousness of wholeness and the qualities of light? There are indeed many ways to do this and every spiritual path has their own way. I will share one way that I have found is the most direct and fastest way to address and connect with your heart and heal. Nonetheless, it is important to keep in mind the nurturing of yourself on all levels is key to continuing the healing that you begin in your heart. It is not a one time shot, it is a process of unfolding throughout your life to listen to your needs and address them as they come up.

The process of healing is to allow these limited qualities that we have taken on throughout our lifetime to transform. With fertility we are usually talking about limited beliefs of unworthiness, being unlovable, feeling insecure with ourselves and our gender, fears, disappointments, despair, helplessness and hopelessness. These qualities are the most common, but we of course are not limited to these in any way. These erroneous beliefs or pictures, as I will refer to them from here on out, are transformed from being a limited picture in our consciousness, to a the essence of light itself. As we do this, we are allowing these limited qualities to transform into virtues of truth; strength, beauty, life essence, peace, love, hope, goodness, worthiness, safety, guidance, wisdom and others and returning to our wholeness within. As these virtues are transformed healing is created on all levels of our being, including the physical body.

It is important to understand that energy, or light as it's referred to, is the underlining force that animates and dictates our existence. This light has various frequencies densities and qualities to it. As it transforms from denser pictures from limiting beliefs to lighter qualities from higher truths, it affects all the subtle levels of our being. This means that it affects our emotional body, our mental body and the physical body. The quality of the light that we are open to determines the bio-chemistry, which in turn affects our glandular and hormonal system, thus having a great impact on our reproductive system as a whole. In conclusion, changes made in the ethereal levels (light levels) move through the denser levels of conscious manifestation and become manifest in the physical levels of our body.

An example of this may be the way we experience stress deteriorating our bodies, or nervousness affecting our stomachs. These are examples as to how the emotions are correlated with the physical body. There really is no separation between these energetic levels, but we create separation in our minds because we are not able to see the more subtle layers of our being. Therefore, we tend to only see and acknowledge the physical. The physical body is the densest and all the other subtle levels are there, just not as visible with our eyes, but perceivable with our emotions, and with our hearts.

Acceptance, Mercy and Letting Go

I used to think of people saying to me" allow the mercy to come in, have mercy for yourself, don't be so hard on yourself" and I really didn't get it. I really didn't get what that meant on a deeper level. I heard the words they would say, and I would think how can I just lay back with this and not do anything about it, that was my interpretation of having acceptance and mercy. In other words, what is it that I am doing that isn't allowing the mercy? I would wonder how would people know that I was being "too hard" on myself and what did that really mean? Should I not strive for what I want, should I just wait for it, where was the balance of those two things and how do I know when I am not being merciful with myself. These are all questions that I would get tangled up in because basically I did not understand that concept and what it meant in my heart.

Consequently, a few weeks later, I had an experience in a healing with a fertility patient who was very angry, who would show me what acceptance and mercy was. This patient was angry at the way she was being treated and she felt left out and abandoned as a child. IN her healing session it was evident the line of pain that her anger at men had caused her throughout her life. Underneath her anger was hurt, the hurt from feeling she did not receive the love she really needed as a child. Underneath that pain was a decision she had made about herself that she wasn't good enough and somehow didn't deserve the love. The fact that she didn't deserve the love was based on the absence of love that was experienced by her from her caregivers in her childhood. Her assumption was "there must be something wrong with me if they are not giving me the love."

As children we usually take on the responsibility and make ourselves wrong for many reasons. One of them is to create safety in our world. We feel safer if our caregivers are right and can guide us in the world, because we are dependant on them and the world is too overwhelming for us to navigate on our own. If we were to know that the adults around us are wrong, then we would feel too unsafe with that adult and therefore, it is easier for us to take on the shame and make ourselves wrong.

Another reason we may blame ourselves, as children, is that most adults imply that children do not know what they are doing or feeling. Caregivers usually imply that children need to learn and this not only creates insecurity and doubt for the children with what they feel and with what they know in their hearts. Automatically, it sets up children as automatically being wrong and taking the blame for any situation. So, again children believe that their feelings can not be trusted and that obviously there is something wrong with them, because their caregivers do not respond the same way.

Nonetheless, this patient now had seen her message of "not good enough" and how she believed that still in her present life right now. She was able to feel the truth, which is that she is completely whole, a perfect reflection of love, peace and is "good enough". This place in her that felt her wound is just that, a wound and not the truth. It was a place where a scared little girl believed a lie, a picture created in her consciousness. She could see how this wounded place in her needed to feel the truth and compassion from the place of her that can see that that was a lie, from the place in her that was standing strong in the truth. But rather than condemning herself for believing that lie (that she wasn't good enough), she was able to see the dynamics that had created it; the caregivers that couldn't give her the love when she needed it, and her own belief due to the circumstances. Once she saw the dynamics that had created her wound and pain, she could now have compassion for herself and understanding from where that came.

The beauty of the forgiveness comes in this case above when she is able to have compassion and understanding of how and why she would feel that way. She can understand that when she felt this wound and unloved in her daily life, in the face of circumstances and other people, she could have mercy for herself instead of judging her self for not being perfect. She could understand that when these feelings of lack of worthiness came up, they were just a part of her past and that understanding would help her see the wholeness that is always there instead of judgment from herself. Now, she was giving herself the mercy from the connection to her deep heart and divine light, learning to parent herself with the love, acceptance and forgiveness she never received. She allowed herself to receive it from her the universal light source through her heart. Instead of getting angry at herself for her feelings, she chose to understand and love herself. And consequently, she became pregnant with her first child and had a healthy baby boy nine months later.

In conclusion, this story shows you how the inner pictures dictate the outer reality of the physical body. Furthermore, it also depicts how to understand our wounds and pictures, and walk through it, so that it doesn't continue to create dysfunction within our physical bodies. It is easy to see how our subjective realities create pictures of lies and how these lies keep us in pain and suffering. On this journey you are learning about many truths that we were not taught to you before and how important it is to embrace these truths of wholeness as it becomes the goal to reach and understand. The road of healing is where we open ourselves up and walk through these painful parts of ourselves and continue to walk to the where we can sit in knowing the Truth of wholeness that we carry.

Clearing of the Pictures
Meditation

1. We offer a prayer of intention: Dear Beloved Divine, please allow me to receive the complete healing for my being, for my body, my mind, my emotions, my heart and my soul. Please fill me with complete light of your Divine qualities and help me to continue to turn towards the Divine light everyday and every minute of my day, amen. I thank you very much for this sacred time you have given me to receive this healing.

2. Now sit quietly and comfortably and begin to notice the chair or bed that is holding you. Begin to allow yourself to fall back into it and let yourself be supported by that chair. Feel the support not just from the chair but also from the Universe around you. Begin to breathe into your body deeply, feeling your body and noticing how your body feels physically…is it tired, heavy, light, tingling, sore, empty, etc…. Take a few minutes…

3. Now, notice your heart and heart area in the upper chest. Breathe into this area primarily. Bring your awareness into your heart area and just feel it for a few minutes. Just feel

your heart. Is there any worries, fears, emptiness, heaviness, confusion, anxiety, depression? Become aware of what you are feeling in this first layer. As you breathe into these emotions or sensations, give them conscious permission to be there. In other words, accept that this is what you are feeling and that as uncomfortable as it may be it is there. Let it be there. Do not fight to change it. Allow yourself to notice it and then allow yourself to breathe deeply allowing the Universal Light to come in and radiate through these places in your heart. Continue to do this for a few minutes, as you naturally allow yourself to move deeper into your heart, by just setting your intention to do so, and knowing that the Universal Light will guide the process where it needs to go.

4. Remember you are not in charge now, all you are doing is saying yes to the Light Essence to direct this process of healing, and there is nothing that you need to change or do or fix. You are just becoming aware of your experience without any judgment of good or bad. You are also observing all resistance and letting it be, all emotions and sensations and letting them be.

5. As you notice these sensations… gently bring breath into them and watch yourself moving deeper into your heart. It's like passing by someone on the train station and you say hello, I acknowledge you, I accept that you are there and I am moving on deeper. You are not necessarily stopping to chat….just in love and kindness acknowledging and moving on.

6. Now, as you continue to move into your deep heart towards your wholeness, you may feel these sensations intensifying, or you may feel a different sensation of feeling, as well as you may see colors or lights or just have a sense of tranquility and peace. Observe what you are feeling and becoming aware of and allow yourself to have that experience without any judgment. Set an intention to bring up whatever is in the way of you having your deepest desire fulfilled in relationship to healing your body and your fertility issues.

7. Once you have put that request in your heart, allow yourself to become aware of what happens. Notice what you feel and start bringing the light into it. Notice if any pictures start to arise… it may look like thoughts from the past, feelings or even scenes from the past that make you feel a certain way.

All these are pictures that are in the way of receiving the highest vibration of light. These pictures are just beliefs, coupled with emotions and experiences of your interpretation of events in your life and the significance you have attached to them. What ultimately happens is that we are able to release the significance and meaning that we have given these events from our lives. We are able to embrace the true meaning and reflection of them in our lives and their higher purpose.

8. As you start to feel what is in your deep heart, bring acceptance to it and then see the light of your breath coming into your deep heart too. Whether you want to relate to that light as Universal Love or Peace, or God… it is nonetheless the highest level of light possible.

9. In many other spiritual paths we use mantras to help break through these pictures. And the ancient languages carry a certain vibration that opens up these subtle energy fields so that they are disbursed into their true form. As a side note it is important to know that the name for God, in ancient languages, is the highest vibration of light there is. Therefore using for example, the name Jesus used for God in Sanskrit; Allaha, or the name of God in the ancient language

of Arabic; Allah, can be powerful, when bringing in the highest vibration of light. You may also use Om, used by the Hindus, meaning the highest vibration of the ultimate reality (God). These are some examples of languages that hold a very high vibration and help to open up the heart energy.

10. Gently repeat the mantra you have chosen, over and over, either out loud or in your mind. It is helpful to say it aloud at the beginning. As you say your mantra, see the light vibration that comes with it, within your breath, moving completely through your body and into the picture that you are experiencing. Continue to breathe this mantra and the light into all the sensations of the pictures, whether they are emotions, thoughts or images. This may continue for 30 minutes or for one hour or longer. Try to continue until the light and the mantra fills your heart completely and you do not feel any more pictures or sensations for the moment.

11. Sit quietly for a few minutes and feel the light and the mantra fill your complete being, connecting with your deep heart and moving into every cell in your body. As this light moves through the pictures, it brings a higher vibration to all the cells and allows the healing. Breathe it in, feel it expand

throughout your being, knowing that this light is greater and more powerful than anything you may have experienced and that it brings truth and all the beautiful qualities of the highest. Also know that this light is able to move through any picture and subjective belief that sit in your consciousness and transform it easily and effortlessly. Our only job is to surrender all our past and our pictures to this light so that we may move past our limitations and pain. By surrendering, I mean allowing yourself to trust the light, to give fully yourself and your pain to this light and watch what happens. Surrendering control is essential in allowing yourself to heal.

12. As you move deeper into your pictures or thoughts with the light, you may experience feelings of fear, disappointment, hopelessness, or others in correlation to your condition at the moment. Know that none of these feelings are truth; they are subjective reality and created by your perception of reality. Allow yourself to suspend these meanings into this light and see what happens.

13. Continue to fill yourself with the light, gently accepting whatever feeling or picture comes up and bringing the light of the mantra into it. Continue to do this until you feel are completely full of the light. Watch the pictures or emotions dissolve into the light. Sit quietly absorbing all these qualities and filling yourself up, drinking from this Divine essence. When you feel ready you may gently open your eyes and slowly reintegrate yourself into your environment.

Judgement and Shame

Thus, with each one of ourselves, we can take the case of our infertility and look at it in the following way: We enter into our doctor's office and the doctor says, "your levels are fine but it is obvious by the fact that you have being trying to conceive unsuccessfully for the past four years, that there is something WRONG with your system, even though it is unexplained." After hearing this word wrong, you start to well up with feelings that are overwhelming. Suddenly, you may feel angry, hurt, disappointed, confused, helpless or all of these. Sometimes you direct all these feelings outside of you, at your doctor, the staff, the place or your husband…or maybe you fall into a deeper state of directing these feeling at yourself.

If you look underneath the overwhelming feelings of defensiveness and blame, there is usually a layer of disappointment and real emotional pain. On a deeper level there is a place that you are judging yourself for having something WRONG, which sounds something like this; "How can I have something WRONG, this will never be fixed, it is hopeless, I am a failure, I am no good, I am worthless and I am unlovable, etc..." Usually the place we go deep inside ourselves in our wound is somewhere where we feel we really don't deserve anything good and where we feel we are failures, unlovable, "wrong", not worthy of conceiving, etc... This is called shame.

In truth, this is our wound. All the events leading to this point have made us look at this wound we carry inside. This is what this event outside of ourselves has made us see and face so that it can be healed. There is another place of wholeness inside that I call the Truth of who we are, but in this moment you are having a reaction from your shame, the place of pain. From the place of wholeness, you can feel the truth, know that you really are worth the love, know that you are the love and know that you are whole. Regardless of how much shame you feel, this wholeness is still there for you and everyone else, it is the essence of who we are. These feelings of pain are all just pictures from your subjective reality that you can feel, believe, and have subscribed to until now, so that you are becoming aware of it.

Commonly we get stuck in that place of feeling the shame and we continue to judge ourselves for it. Even when we understand the pattern of our wound, we may start to feel impatient and hopeless. This place of impatience is not able to experience acceptance, compassion or mercy for ourselves. In essence, we are still in a place of judgment for ourselves because we just want to finish feeling our discomfort and not feel the pain anymore.

These deep places of shame and judgment can be frightening and painful, especially because most of us did not receive the love unconditionally from our parents or caregivers and somewhere along the line it hurt us deeply. We have built our whole lives over that wound of feeling wrong (shame) and those contributing beliefs. So when we start to unravel them it may seem like too much pain to bear and too overwhelming, but the truth is that we are creating our lives over this pain, feeling the deep level of dissatisfaction in our being and trying to ignore it. This deep level of dissatisfaction penetrates through everything in our lives and completely affects our physiology, until we decide to face it and heal it.

Living with this deep level of dissatisfaction in our lives is, in my experience, more painful than going through these wounds and dispelling the false beliefs. In moving towards our wholeness, we can see that there is a problem because we haven't been successful at conceiving, but this problem does not determine your self worth. If your tubes are blocked, it does not determine how good of a person you are, or if you could be a good mother. It does not mean that you are being punished because you are essentially bad. It has no correlation with your worth.

We all have the ability to feel the wholeness of our being in our hearts. Our worth is who we are, whole and complete, not who we attached meaning to on the outer. Many of us identify our being and our worth with what we do outside in the world and with what we have acquired. We are all essence of the divine, spiritual in nature and carry that spirituality in our hearts. Our worth is all worthy, and our hearts are our bridge to our spirit and to the Divine wholeness.

In our humanity we are not taught this wholeness as an experience rather as an intellectual concept, and not as a practical reality. In our culture we continue to identify with our outside actions and achievements to determine our worth. The truth is as spiritual beings, our worth is greater than we could ever single-handedly achieve in this lifetime. Our worth is greater than all the physical riches in this world. The richness is truly within us in our hearts.

In turn, we must release the judgment that we feel in our hearts and accept that these wounds are there, and that no matter how strong the shame feels it isn't really real, it is just the level of consciousness we have been living in. Having acceptance and understanding of where these come from, and where our pain comes from allows us to unravel them and break free from their control. It allows us to enter into a higher level of consciousness where our bodies are whole and not affected physiologically.

Shame also makes us feel that we do not deserve any of our deepest desires; because of course we are not worthy (would be one of the voices of shame). For many, many generations we have been taught that desire is bad and there is a mass consciousness of shame around women in general. It is your typical mass consciousness religious conservative view that desire or even enjoyment is wrong and that it is the seat of many evils in the world. So, many of us have turned that view towards all desire that we may have. Although the greed and selfish pursuit of desire may lead to destruction and many other negative outcomes in our world, surely we are not talking about that kind of greed. When we feel the yearning within ourselves to want a child, to love a child, to nurture a child we may think that this may be selfish of ourselves and blame ourselves for desiring such. Besides the voice of shame may say, "There are many children in the world that need a home and I shouldn't be wanting my own". Another voice of shame may say, "we are not worthy to ask for what God has not given us, that in fact if God has not given us this "gift" then there may be a reason why and that perhaps it is better to "not ask for what I want but settle for what God has given me." Even though there is some truth to that statement about acceptance of what has been given to us at each moment, there is also some twisted blaming and shaming going on, in the background.

It is important to recognize our voices of shame that lay deep in our hearts and turn them also to the light. This voice of shame is just a picture that was created throughout your lifetime and lodged as consciousness in your being. From our place of wholeness, all of us are worthy of asking for and wanting to conceive. We can also include personal desires of having a baby, of wanting and deserving a baby. This desire is not wrong in any way.

Perhaps there could be a reason for not having had the child just yet, but this reason is not correlated to your feelings of unworthiness, nor to whether you deserve this child or not. The truth is we don't know what the reason is, but just the same we can't assume that because it hasn't happened that it's not going to either. Rather, unraveling the underlying beliefs is one way that we may shift our consciousness and heal whatever issues are contributing to our present condition in our bodies.

Many of us women have ingrained in our consciousness the belief that it is wrong to have needs, to have desire and to feel good about ourselves. We have been fed the image of the sacrificial wife, mother, daughter, always putting other's needs before our own. While a life of service is honorable, there is a way in which if taken to the extreme, or out of balance with our own caring for ourselves, actually depletes our own resources and weakens our body, mind and spirit, leaving us extremely vulnerable to disease and disorders. This cultural belief creates difficulty when we have strong desires for a family and it doesn't become a reality.

We may begin to question those desires. We may start to feel guilt for having these desires, having thoughts that resonate to this; "After all, there are so many children in the world that need parents, maybe it is wrong for us to want this", and so on and so forth. It is easy for us to start to feel guilt and undeserving and fall into the rut of feeling that our needs and desires are superficial and somewhat shame based overall, and not deserving of our attention.

The shameful feelings that are around any desire that we have are closely intertwined with our feeling of self worth again. As women a large part of our consciousness has been ingrained with the feeling of shame for our bodies, our sexuality and with any desire. This shame that extends from just being female is extended to having desires, and therefore makes desires just as unacceptable as being female. So, immediately desires of any kind become linked with shame, and we constantly haunt ourselves with this shame based feelings that have been passed on through centuries of generations.

Women have fought a long history with the battle of conflict of desire and shame of our bodies and being. Our bodies have always taken a shame based position and many of us have accepted this shame as truth and kept it well hidden, within ourselves.

Our body carries the dance of life that we were designed with. It is not something that has to be made wrong in order to be "good enough". It is by design that we have feelings and desires and all of it is part of being a female. It is by the design of that dance of attraction that life continues, and we procreate. Our sexuality is the way the Divine essence works through us to procreate. Our body is our vessel in which life transforms itself from essence to form. Our body is beautiful within itself. It is a gift, the gift of life. Our body is not intended to be a vessel for shame and disgust; it is a beautiful vessel of creation. The truth is that women are the vessels of our humanity that have the gift of cultivating life while seeded with the masculine energy.

The creation of man and woman is holy. It comes from perfect divinity. Our bodies are holy and have a gift of allowing life to come through and continue creation. When we recognize this truth about who we are, we are able to slowly let go of the imposing images of shame that we have been handed down through generations.

Holding on to these feelings of shame and limitations of our bodies and our own essence continues to create dis-ease in our bodies, and it can affect our hormones, our reproductive system and our fertility. It is important to really understand and see ourselves in the wholeness that we were created. And in this same light, it is important to also see that our life is steeped in goodness and in divine wisdom.

Being responsible with ourselves and taking care of our needs and respecting our desires are crucial in fulfilling ourselves. We were created to experience joy and happiness in our hearts, and moving towards this in our life is part of the divine flow of life. Life is about being happy, even if we don't get everything that we want, when we want it. But moving in that direction and realizing that living is joyous and doesn't have to be all about struggle and suffering, is crucial to fulfilling our hearts and souls.

It is our responsibility to move from struggle and suffering to fulfillment. First, we must realize our wholeness is a source of joy, peace and love that is constantly there within us and all around us. Secondly, we deserve happiness, and finally, it our responsibility to ourselves to fulfill that for ourselves with, of course, our reliance on the universal light Consciousness that supports us all. And it is still our responsibility to fulfill our desires, to follow our deepest hearts inspiration and to take care of ourselves out of love. This includes caring enough for ourselves to take good proper care, to eat nourishing foods, to move our bodies, to take time out when we need it, to do things we enjoy, to laugh, to play, to sing and dance and to listen deeply to our own hearts.

Therefore, part of healing is being able to let go of our shame and see our bodies, our sexuality and our role as women as the holy role that it is. It is important to accept that feeling good and wanting to feel good about ourselves is sacred and in alignment with the universal light consciousness. It is not wrong in any way and seeking what you desire in life is in alignment with higher source.

In conclusion I want you to take a few minutes to really feel the divine gift of being a female and what that intention of that Feminine Wisdom really is, what a beautiful gift you have been given in this body. Even if your body is not producing or creating now, try to connect with the fact that you are a woman and that this in itself is a gift that you have been given. Even if you do not understand at the moment why you are experiencing these problems, try to see yourself as your deeper truth of a sacred creation of the Divine and sit with that while you breathe in deeply, regardless of what imbalance you may be experiencing temporarily.

Our Feminine Body as the Vessel of Creation Meditation

1. Sit comfortably in a quiet place where you will not be disturbed for a few minutes. Bring your attention deep into your body and scan your body. Become aware of what you are feeling. Where are you holding tension, where is your body loose and comfortable? Where are you feeling pressure or any other sensation? Notice your breathing... is it fast or slow... does it feel rushed or anxious? Connect with your breathing... acknowledging that it contains the Divine light consciousness and it moves through your whole being, bringing light and life. Take a few minutes to focus on your breathing... let it permeate through your body, gently softening any areas of tension, allowing you to relax deeper and deeper.

2. As you relax deeper, focus on your chest and heart area. Ask the divine light consciousness to help you to move deeper into the layers of your heart, and to open to receive this light consciousness. Then continue to connect to your breath as it continues to move through you, your heart and your body.

3. Feel the breath expanding within you, this is the time to start using a mantra of the highest vibration; as was discussed before of ALLA HA (word for God used by Jesus in Arameic) or ALLAH (word for God in Arabic) or OM (word for the highest vibration of reality used by the Hindus).

4. Choose your mantra and begin bringing the name into your heart… with each breath that you take… see the name moving through into your heart. Continue this for a few minutes.

5. Then begin to see your breath and the name going into every cell in your body. Moving especially through the whole reproductive area and the pelvic area, bringing light and renewal and love to each and every cell. Allow yourself to accept this new creation that the divine light consciousness is giving you and continue to surrender and trust this light and what you are receiving.

6. See your female body as the vessel for the creation of life. See your uterus as the sacred vessel where life begins and a cell is transformed to grow and grow and grow into a miracle child. As you continue with your mantra and your breath, you are allowing this divine light consciousness to permeate

this reality into your being and your body. Breathe in the wholeness into your pelvic area and know that it exists there and each cell is capable of returning to this wholeness.

7. See the light consciousness filling up this whole area in your pelvis... moving through the uterus... the fallopian tubes... the ovaries.... the spaces in between...and feel the sacredness of wholeness that was created in your body.

8. Your FEMININE BODY is holy, it carries the blueprint of the vessel which allows life to be born and cultivated on our planet. It is the perfect form for the vessel of creation. Feel the gratitude in your heart for having this body and allow the gentle caring for your body to come through. Feel the joy of having this body as a gift... and allow yourself to see yourself as a positive and special part of creation. Let these feelings expand through your heart and through every single cell in your body, including your pelvic area. Conclude by repeating your mantra for another 5 to 10 minutes while you allow all these new levels of consciousness to integrate into your body, mind and soul.

The Jewel Within

"The Woman Contains Everything
And You Say She is The Real Ocean For Everything
She Has
If She Knows Herself"

Shaykh Sidi Muhammad Sa'id Al-Jamal ar-Rifai as-Shadhuli

The Jewel Meditation was created to allow you to sit with yourself and feel the essence of your wholeness and the beautiful jewel of that essence that each one of you carry. By feeling this essence it becomes part of your consciousness and becomes part of your knowing. It becomes easier and easier to live from a place of peace and health rather than from the place of pain and disease. Read this meditation daily if possible and allow yourself the time to heal.

Jewel Meditation

1. Take a seat and relax for a few minutes, breathing gently in and out.... Allow your breath to travel throughout your whole body. Breathing in... breathing out.... Breathing in.... breathing out.... Allow yourself to sink deeper into your heart, into your body, into the chair that you are sitting on. Breathing gently in... and breathing gently out.... Notice how your breathing starts to slow down and settle within your own being. Allow your awareness to focus on your body, how it feels....where there's tension... where there is relaxation... let the breath take you on a journey to explore your jewel.

2. Next as you stay in remembrance, allow your awareness to travel deeper into your body, feeling primarily your heart area and the depth that there is there. Let your heart expand as you focus all your attention into this area. Let the Universal Light start to come in with your breath, directing your attention to a place deeper in your heart. Allow this light to fulfill every single cell in your body. Breathing in... and breathing out.

3. As you let yourself sink even deeper into your body and your heart… you start to move closer to a bright shining light within your being… and curiously you gently allowing yourself to move in closer and closer.

4. As you notice this light within your being… you notice it has many colors of light within it and radiates outwardly, stunningly and brightly.   You start to approach it and you feel a sensation of peace and safety and warmth all coming towards you, enveloping you like a soft fluffy cloud. Your body starts to relax as you feel safer and safer… You begin to dissolve your boundaries and surrender gently to this light within… feeling safe and peaceful. The feeling of peacefulness becomes stronger and stronger… emanating from this powerful light within.

5. You start to notice that this light within your being is yourself and that there are no boundaries between this light and yourself…Your perception of you dissolves into the beautiful radiating light of your being and you feel ecstatic, full of joy and radiant.

6. Now take a few minutes to feel all the qualities that are in this deepest part of your being… the qualities that the

Universal Source has placed deep inside your jewel. This is your jewel and your treasure. This is the essence of your wholeness. Allow yourself to feel your particular colors and qualities that have been placed inside and that are now ready to emanate fully outward and become your conscious reality.

7. There may be qualities of joy, happiness, safety, security, protection, beauty, goodness, unconditional love, compassion, acceptance, forgiveness, understanding, trust, ease, reliance, hope, creation and complete surrender.

8. Feel the lights of each one of these qualities as they penetrate each cell in your body and in your being. Allow then to move through you breaking all the illusional boundaries and become one with your jewel.

9. Bring the remembrance into your breath and allow yourself to expand into this consciousness…. gently and softly, with complete surrender to this truth.

10. Know that this jewel inside yourself is your wholeness; it has been there from the beginning and it will continue. It is our source of life and life essence. It does not change. The only thing that changes is our perception of it and ourselves. The

more awareness we have of it, the more we are able to live in this consciousness, free of pain and suffering. Aspire to explore your essence of your jewel and value what you have been given: the life, the essence, the beauty of being a vessel for the creation of humanity, entrusted with all the qualities within your hidden treasure of your jewel.

"You Are A Treasure Waiting To Be Discovered"

Shaykh Sidi Muhammad Sa'id Al-Jamal ar-Rifai as-Shadhuli

www.ingramcontent.com/pod-product-compliance
Lightning Source LLC
Chambersburg PA
CBHW031151270326
41931CB00006B/222